About the Authors

Pearl B. Werfel, PhD, is a clinical psychologist in private practice in San Francisco. She has been inducted into the National Multiple Sclerosis Society (NMSS) Hall of Fame for Healthcare Professionals and is recognized by them as a trainer for mental health professionals. Dr. Werfel sits on the Healthcare Advisory Committee of the Northern California Chapter of the NMSS and has led numerous workshops for that chapter. She developed an online program for pain and stress management for people with MS and co-developed a class on MS for graduate-level clinical psychology students.

Ron E. Franco Durán, PhD, is a health psychologist and the system-wide Associate Provost for Research and Scholarship at Alliant International University. He has over 30 years of clinical research experience working with persons living with chronic and life-threatening conditions. He has served on the Hispanic/Latino Advisory Board for the NMSS for the past decade, and for the past 4 years he has served on the NMSS Committee for Diversity and Inclusion.

Linda J. Trettin, PhD, is a clinical neuropsychologist with the Mercy General Hospital, Dignity Health and the MS Achievement Center. She obtained certification through the Consortium of Multiple Sclerosis Centers as a Multiple Sclerosis Certified Specialist. Dr. Trettin enjoys collaborating within an interdisciplinary team and leads NMSS-sponsored behavioral health programs.

Advances in Psychotherapy – Evidence-Based Practice

Series Editor
Danny Wedding, PhD, MPH, School of Medicine, American University of Antigua, St. Georges, Antigua

Associate Editors
Larry Beutler, PhD, Professor, Palo Alto University / Pacific Graduate School of Psychology, Palo Alto, CA

Kenneth E. Freedland, PhD, Professor of Psychiatry and Psychology, Washington University School of Medicine, St. Louis, MO

Linda C. Sobell, PhD, ABPP, Professor, Center for Psychological Studies, Nova Southeastern University, Ft. Lauderdale, FL

David A. Wolfe, PhD, RBC Chair in Children's Mental Health, Centre for Addiction and Mental Health, University of Toronto, ON

The basic objective of this series is to provide therapists with practical, evidence-based treatment guidance for the most common disorders seen in clinical practice – and to do so in a reader-friendly manner. Each book in the series is both a compact "how-to" reference on a particular disorder for use by professional clinicians in their daily work and an ideal educational resource for students as well as for practice-oriented continuing education.

The most important feature of the books is that they are practical and easy to use: All are structured similarly and all provide a compact and easy-to-follow guide to all aspects that are relevant in real-life practice. Tables, boxed clinical "pearls," marginal notes, and summary boxes assist orientation, while checklists provide tools for use in daily practice.

Multiple Sclerosis

Pearl B. Werfel
Private Practice, San Francisco, CA

Ron E. Franco Durán
Alliant International University, Los Angeles, CA

Linda J. Trettin
Mercy General Hospital, Dignity Health, Sacramento, CA and
MS Achievement Center, Citrus Heights, CA

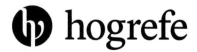

Library of Congress Cataloging in Publication information for the print version of this book is available via the Library of Congress Marc Database under the Library of Congress Control Number 2015956012

Library and Archives Canada Cataloguing in Publication
Werfel, Pearl B., author
       Multiple sclerosis / Pearl B. Werfel (Private Practice, San Francisco, CA), Ron E. Franco Durán (Alliant International University, Los Angeles, CA), Linda J. Trettin (Mercy General Hospital, Dignity Health, Sacramento, CA, and MS Achievement Center, Citrus Heights, CA).

(Advances in psychotherapy--evidence-based practice ; volume 36)
Includes bibliographical references.
Issued in print and electronic formats.
ISBN 978-0-88937-409-6 (paperback).--ISBN 978-1-61676-409-8 (pdf).--
ISBN 978-1-61334-409-5 (html)

       1. Multiple sclerosis. 2. Multiple sclerosis--Diagnosis. 3. Multiple sclerosis--Treatment. I. Franco Durán, Ron E., author II. Trettin, Linda J., author III. Title. IV. Series: Advances in psychotherapy--evidence-based practice ; v. 36

RC377.W37 2016   616.8'34   C2015-908127-0
                                          C2015-908128-9

Cover image © fotolia.com/styf

© 2016 by Hogrefe Publishing
http://www.hogrefe.com

PUBLISHING OFFICES
USA: Hogrefe Publishing Corporation, 38 Chauncy Street, Suite 1002, Boston, MA 02111
                  Phone (866) 823-4726, Fax (617) 354-6875; E-mail customerservice@hogrefe.com
EUROPE: Hogrefe Publishing GmbH, Merkelstr. 3, 37085 Göttingen, Germany
                  Phone +49 551 99950-0, Fax +49 551 99950-111; E-mail publishing@hogrefe.com

SALES & DISTRIBUTION
USA: Hogrefe Publishing, Customer Services Department,
                  30 Amberwood Parkway, Ashland, OH 44805
                  Phone (800) 228-3749, Fax (419) 281-6883; E-mail customerservice@hogrefe.com
UK: Hogrefe Publishing, c/o Marston Book Services Ltd., 160 Eastern Ave.,
                  Milton Park, Abingdon, OX14 4SB, UK
                  Phone +44 1235 465577, Fax +44 1235 465556; E-mail direct.orders@marston.co.uk
EUROPE: Hogrefe Publishing, Merkelstr. 3, 37085 Göttingen, Germany
                  Phone +49 551 99950-0, Fax +49 551 99950-111; E-mail publishing@hogrefe.com

OTHER OFFICES
CANADA: Hogrefe Publishing, 660 Eglinton Ave. East, Suite 119-514, Toronto, Ontario, M4G 2K2
SWITZERLAND: Hogrefe Publishing, Länggass-Strasse 76, CH-3000 Bern 9

Hogrefe Publishing
Incorporated and registered in the Commonwealth of Massachusetts, USA, and in Göttingen, Lower Saxony, Germany

Printed and bound in the USA

ISBN 978-0-88937-409-6 (print) • ISBN 978-1-61676-409-8 (PDF) • ISBN 978-1-61334-409-5 (EPUB)
http://doi.org/10.1027/00409-000

Preface

Multiple sclerosis (MS) is a complex, unpredictable, and chronic neurologic disorder that can affect numerous bodily systems. There is no known cause or cure. The disease process can result in minimal symptoms or significant disability. The cover photograph illustrates the precarious nature of MS; while at one point the disease can appear to be stable, at another point, symptoms and functioning can change and successful interventions can become less effective. The role of the mental health professional has been well recognized in evidenced-based treatment of individuals living with MS. Indeed, mental health providers interface with individuals living with MS across the course of the disorder.

There is no definitive medical or psychological MS theory or treatment. However, the trend in healthcare is toward integrative medicine, and the National MS Society and the Consortium of Multiple Sclerosis Centers both recognize the importance of comprehensive care for people living with MS. Numerous professionals may be part of an MS treatment team, and each team member may have its own perspective, research, and terminology. We will be drawing on research from many fields in an attempt to highlight both the challenges and the resources available for someone who is living with MS and those who provide support.

The following abbreviations are used frequently throughout the book:

CID   Chronic illness and disability
CNS   Central nervous system
DMTs   Disease-modifying treatments
DSM-5   *Diagnostic and Statistical Manual of Mental Disorders*, Fifth Edition
MS   Multiple sclerosis
NMSS   National Multiple Sclerosis Society
PPMS   Primary progressive multiple sclerosis
PRMS   Progressive–relapsing multiple sclerosis
RRMS   Relapsing–remitting multiple sclerosis
SPMS   Secondary progressive multiple sclerosis

Acknowledgments

The authors have been blessed with the ability to join with colleagues whom we enjoy and respect, to grow together and create something that will help others. We are grateful to the editors for this rare opportunity, and we especially want to thank Dr. Danny Wedding for all of his support and encouragement. Many people have offered their expertise and encouragement during this project. We wish to thank Dr. Shelley Peery for consultation and editing; Sheila Kolenc for layout and technical assistance; Dr. John A. Schafer and Dr. Sabeen Lulu for contributing their knowledge on MS; Dr. Rhoda Olkin for consultation on disability; and Dr. Rosalind Kalb, Jaclyn Smoczynski, and Janelle Del Carlo of the NMSS for their assistance and encouragement.

Dedication

This book is dedicated to people who live with MS and those who help and support them. A portion of the proceeds of this book will be donated to the National Multiple Sclerosis Society.

Table of Contents

1

Description

1.1   Terminology

A working knowledge of terminology related to multiple sclerosis (MS) is important. Multiple domains of an individual's life can be touched by MS, and the disease poses various challenges. A comprehensive understanding of related terms facilitates effective communication with other healthcare providers, informs the education provided to individuals with MS, and aids the clinician's formulation of a comprehensive treatment plan. Tables 1, 2, 3, and 4 provide an overview of relevant terminology associated with biopsychosocial factors that may impact the life of a person with MS. In addition, more detailed and inclusive overviews of MS-related terminology and definitions are available from the National Multiple Sclerosis Society (NMSS; http://www.nationalmssociety.org) and the Consortium of Multiple Sclerosis Centers (http://www.mscare.org).

Table 1
MS-Specific Terminology

Term	Definition
Multiple sclerosis	An unpredictable disease of the central nervous system (CNS) that disrupts the flow of information within the brain, and between the brain and body (NMSS; http://www.nationalmssociety.org/what-is-MS); four disease courses have been identified (Lublin & Reingold, 1996).
Relapsing–remitting course	Episodes of acute worsening of neurologic function, with some amount of recovery and no progression in between.
Secondary progressive course	Following an initial relapsing–remitting course, the disease transitions in many people to a steadily progressive form with increased loss of function.
Primary progressive course	Continuing worsening of disease from onset, without distinct relapses.
Progressive relapsing course	Progressive disease from onset, with occasional acute relapses and continuing disease progression.

Table 1 (continued)

Term	Definition
Clinically isolated syndrome	A temporary diagnosis that may initially be given if insufficient brain magnetic resonance imaging (MRI) evidence is present at first clinical presentation. Implies increased risk for future confirmed MS, given the need for subsequent evidence of further clinical relapses or new MRI lesions.
Radiologically isolated syndrome (RIS)	MRI abnormalities typical of CNS demyelination in the absence of clinical symptoms; treatment/diagnosis made on a case-by-case basis or after exam findings suggestive of demyelinating events.

Table 2
Relevant Biological and Neurological Terminology

Term	Definition
Antigen	Any substance that causes your immune system to produce antibodies against it. An antigen may be a foreign substance from the environment (e.g., chemicals, bacteria, viruses, or pollen) or formed within the body (e.g., bacterial toxins or tissue cells).
Autoimmunity; autoimmune disease; immune-mediated disease	The prefix *auto* means *self* — that is, the immune system is reacting against normally occurring antigens in the body, as if these antigens were foreign (NMSS).
Axon	Also known as nerve fiber; the extension of the cell body that carries messages (NMSS).
Axonal (also, dendritic) sprouting	A phenomenon in which injured axons regenerate or "sprout" new terminal connections (Loring, 1999).
Blood–brain barrier (BBB)	A semi-permeable barrier that excludes many chemicals in the blood from entering the cerebrospinal fluid (CSF) and brain. This barrier is not absolute. The probable functions of the BBB include exclusion of blood-borne toxic substances and protection from systemic neurotransmitters and hormones (Loring, 1999).
CNS	Brain and spinal cord.
Cerebral spinal fluid (CSF)	Fluid produced in the choroid plexus that serves as a protective hydraulic system to cushion the brain and spinal cord from jarring injury. CSF may be examined as part of a neurological work-up because many CSF alterations may reflect nervous system impairment. Samples of CSF are obtained by lumbar puncture (Loring, 1999), and analysis of CSF is helpful in the diagnosis of MS.

Table 2 (continued)

Term	Definition
Cortex, cerebral	Outer layer of the brain consisting of gray matter. Its surface area is greatly increased by being folded into convolutions called *gyri*, which are separated by furrows, or grooves, called *sulci* (Loring, 1999).
Cranial nerves	Twelve paired nerves arising from the brain stem that innervate muscles of the head and receive sensory information, primarily from the head (Loring, 1999).
Demyelination	Destruction of the myelin sheath surrounding a nerve fiber that disrupts neural conduction. The most common demyelinating disease is MS (Loring, 1999).
Disease-modifying treatments	Medications prescribed to modify the disease course.
Gadolinium	A chemical compound given during MRI scans that helps distinguish new lesions from old lesions.
Immunoglobulin G (IgG)	An antibody-containing substance produced by human plasma cells in diseased CNS plaques. Levels of IgG are often increased in the CSF in patients with MS.
Lhermitte's sign	The radiation of tingling or electric-like paresthesias into the limbs or trunk on flexion of the neck.
Myelin sheath	The fatty insulating substance surrounding nerve fibers in the white matter of the brain and spinal cord (NMSS).
Neurodegenerative	Disease process that reflects the progressive loss of structure or function of neurons, including death of neurons.
Oligodendrocytes	Cells that make and maintain myelin.
Optic neuritis	An inflammatory disorder of the optic nerve that commonly occurs in only one eye and causes visual loss and sometimes blindness; it is usually temporary.
Paresthesias	Abnormal sensations such as numbness, prickling, or "pins and needles."
Peripheral nervous system (PNS)	Nerves and axons that connect the CNS to muscles, sensory organs, and glands
Plaques (lesions)	Scarring (also called lesions).
Relapses	Random attacks of inflammation. Also known as exacerbations or flare-ups.
Spasticity	Involuntary muscle contractions leading to spasms and stiffness or rigidity (primarily affecting the lower limbs in MS).
T cells	T cells, which are one type of white blood cell in the immune system, somehow become sensitized to proteins

Table 2 (continued)

Term	Definition
	in the CNS. When T cells become activated, they enter the CNS through blood vessels and produce damaging inflammation. Once in the CNS, these T cells not only injure myelin, but also secrete chemicals that damage nerve fibers (axons) and recruit more damaging immune cells to the site of inflammation.
Transverse myelitis	An acute spinal cord disorder causing sudden low back pain as well as muscle weakness and abnormal sensory sensations in the lower extremities.
White matter	A component of the CNS in the brain and superficial spinal cord. White matter consists mostly of glial cells (i.e., cells that form myelin, and provide support and protection for neurons) and myelinated axons that transmit signals from one region to another. While *gray matter* is primarily associated with processing and cognition, white matter modulates the distribution of action potentials, acting as a relay and coordinating communication between different brain regions.

Table 3
Cognitive and Neuropsychological Terminology

Term	Definition
Cognition	Mental processes associated with attention, perception, thinking, learning, and memory (Loring, 1999).
Delirium	A temporary and usually reversible confusional state involving alterations in level of arousal, disturbances of attention, and impairment in the logical stream of thought. Onset is rapid, with a fluctuating course (Loring, 1999).
Dementia	An umbrella term used to reflect the fact that cognitive dysfunction has resulted in impairment in independent living.
Neuropsychiatric; neurobehavioral	Describes mental disorders, as well as affective and behavioral symptoms, that can be attributed to diseases of the nervous system.

Table 4
Rehabilitation Terminology

Term	Definition
Rehabilitation	Neurorehabilitation aims to aid recovery from a nervous system injury/disease and to minimize and/or compensate for any functional disturbances (e.g., activities of daily living, communication, mobility). Rehabilitation specialists include an interdisciplinary team of speech, physical, and occupational therapists, as well as psychologists and physicians.
Impairments	Refers to the symptoms and limitations caused directly by CNS damage (e.g., decreased vision, decreased strength, spasticity, tremor, etc.)
Disability	Refers to the reduction in function in the performance of tasks (e.g., walking, bathing, etc.).
Handicap	Refers to the reduced ability to participate in various life situations (e.g., driving, employment, etc.) and the environmental restrictions that the patient suffers.
Remediation	Correcting the problem. This restorative approach consists of reinforcing previously learned patterns of behavior (Loring, 1999).
Compensation	An alternative means of task performance because the preferred approach has become more difficult or impossible secondary to impairment or disability. Also, modifying the environment or use of assistive devices to accommodate changes.

1.1.1 Psychiatric Disorders and Psychosocial Problems Associated With MS

Mental health professionals often find it useful to distinguish between psychosocial problems encountered by many individual living with MS and comorbid psychiatric disorders. Such a distinction can aid in the comprehensive conceptualization of the individual and treatment formulation. Psychosocial problems, which reflect psychological, interpersonal, and social adjustment difficulties, may be faced by individuals prior to definitive diagnosis of MS, as well as throughout various stages of the course of MS. Psychiatric disorders are defined by the classification system within the fifth edition of the *Diagnostic and Statistical Manual of Mental Disorders* (DSM-5; American Psychiatric Association, 2013) and the *International Statistical Classification of Diseases and Related Health Problems* (ICD-10; World Health Organization, 2007) and can also appear prior to or subsequent to the diagnosis of MS.

1.1.2   Psychiatric Diagnoses Associated With MS

Mental health professionals have an important place in the management of MS. Common symptoms associated with MS that are amenable to psychological intervention include mood disorders, cognitive disorders, adjustment disorders, interpersonal difficulties, and potential neurobehavioral symptoms associated with neurologic disease and medication effects.

Potentially relevant comorbid psychiatric diagnoses that mental health professionals may use to classify clinically significant problems are based on the DSM-5 (American Psychiatric Association, 2013). Table 5 shows diagnoses that may be encountered within a clinical setting while working with individuals with MS. Given the variability of diagnostic codes for select disorders listed in Table 5, the reader is referred to the DSM-5 for further detail.

Table 5
Psychiatric Diagnoses Associated With MS

Mood disorders	DSM-5 (ICD-10)
Major depressive disorder	296.99 (F34.8)
Adjustment disorder with depressed mood	309.0 (F43.21)
Persistent depressive disorder (dysthymia)	300.4 (F34.1)
Depressive disorder due to another medical condition	See DSM-5
Substance/medication-induced depressive disorder	See DSM-5
Bipolar (I or II) disorder (coding depends on severity and whether the most recent episode was manic or depressed)	296.89 (F31.81)
Pseudobulbar affect	F48.2
Cyclothymic disorder	301.13 (F34.0)
Disruptive mood dysregulation disorder	296.99 (F34.8)
Anxiety disorders	**DSM-5 (ICD-10)**
Generalized anxiety disorder	300.02 (F41.1)
Adjustment disorder with anxiety	309.24 (F43.22)
Unspecified anxiety disorder	300 (F41.9)
Anxiety disorder due to another medical condition	293.84 (F06.4)
Substance/medication-induced anxiety disorder	See DSM-5
Somatic symptom disorder or illness anxiety disorder	300.7 (F45.21)
Social anxiety disorder (social phobia)	300.23 (F40.10)
Agoraphobia; also see panic disorder	300.01 (F41.0)
Specific phobia (e.g., needle/injection phobia)	See DSM-5

Table 5 (continued)

Personality	DSM-5 (ICD-10)
Personality change due to another medical condition	310.1 (F07.0)
Personality disorders	301.83 (F60.3)
Personality change as an associated feature in delirium	See DSM-5
Personality change as an associated feature of major or mild neurocognitive disorder	See DSM-5
Personality change as a result of a substance use disorder	See DSM-5
Psychological factors affecting other medical conditions	316 (F54)
Cognitive disorders	DSM-5 (ICD-10)
Major or mild neurocognitive disorder due to another medical condition	See DSM-5

1.1.3   Psychosocial Problems Associated With MS

Corbin and Strauss (1988) wrote:

> When a severe chronic illness comes crashing into someone's life, it cannot help but separate the person of the present from the person of the past and affect or even shatter any images of self held for the future. Unless the illness is mild or its effects on activity are relatively negligible, who I was in the past and hope to be in the future are rendered discontinuous with who I am in the present. New conceptions of who and what I am – past, present, and future – must arise out of what remains. (p. 10)

Often, individuals are faced with adjusting their self-image from invulnerable or healthy to one that includes living with a chronic illness. Psychosocial consequences can influence numerous areas of life, with distress related to disruptions to life goals, employment, finances, independence, relationships, and activities of daily living (Mohr et al., 1999). A change in self-image may arise from any aspect of MS, such as incontinence, sexual dysfunction, reduced mobility, or cognitive problems. Therapists can explore why the changed and/or lost abilities were important and identify alternative methods to meet those needs.

While self-image refers to how one thinks about himself/herself, stigma reflects others' views of an individual. Reactions from others range from avoidance to being overly solicitous. However, stigma should be differentiated from difficulties clients have in their own self-image that are projected onto others; these assumptions of how others view or will treat them may derive from the client's own experiences and attitudes about disability, impairments, and disease prior to the diagnosis of MS. Still, individuals within one's support system may misattribute the root cause of a symptom; for instance, fatigue may be incorrectly identified as "laziness." Anger and frustration can develop

Covert symptoms (fatigue, pain, cognitive dysfunction) can be disabling but not visible to others

when the client is invalidated in his or her attempt to describe the impact of their symptoms to others. For instance, when explaining that they are not able participate in planned activities secondary to MS-related fatigue, others may say, "I had a busy day, too" or "I didn't sleep well last night, either." Similarly, clients may hear, "But you look so good," which gives an implicit message that they are not measuring up to expectation. To follow, some symptoms are referred to as "invisible" because they are not readily apparent to others. Some examples of "invisible symptoms" include vision disturbance, fatigue, weakness, pain, prickly or tingling sensations, heat sensitivity, dizziness, and cognitive difficulties. Alternatively, others may assume that limitations exist when there is actually no evidence to support such a conclusion. Moreover, despite legal protections, clients can be vulnerable to discrimination, such as in the work environment.

Identity issues may include self-doubt, self-criticism, and the loss of one's sense of current skills and future capabilities

Social role and relationship difficulties in MS are associated with lack of social support, isolation, and social withdrawal. In an effort to regain a sense of control over an unpredictable disease process and maintain independence, individuals can refuse help from others. Alternatively, dependency issues can develop in multiple facets of relationships, including emotional, physical, medical, and financial spheres. Within relationships, the client can experience fear of abandonment. Such fear can underlie isolation, or trigger other potential destructive behaviors that are detrimental to the relationship. For clients who are not in a relationship, uncertainty about dating and meeting a life partner is common.

Low levels of social support in MS have been shown to be associated with depression

Individuals may avoid talking to family and friends about their MS. Avoidance may stem from a fear of potentially burdening others, causing others to worry, or concern that they will be treated differently than they were prior to having MS. Relevant related psychosocial issues may include intimacy, communication, division of labor within the family, disclosure of diagnosis to others, community involvement, self-esteem, and independence. Maintaining social ties often requires new methods of approaching relationships wherein the client may learn to become more open with others about the effect of the disease and potential ways MS can affect a relationship. When faced with the prospect of having to cope with a long-term illness, the entire family system may find its usual way of functioning to be challenged.

Fatigue, depression, and cognitive dysfunction have been shown to be major determinants of quality of life in MS

A relevant dimension of psychosocial functioning is quality of life. Quality of life is a multidimensional concept related to individuals' perception of their general well-being and level of role fulfillment across a range of different psychosocial, physical, and symptom-related phenomena. Individuals diagnosed with MS assess their quality of life as reduced compared with the general population and also lower than other chronic disease populations. Multiple challenges to both physical and psychological well-being are often present, as the person may encounter unpleasant and unpredictable symptoms, difficult treatment regimens and drug side effects, and increasing levels of physical disability. The quality of life of individuals with MS has been measured in terms of physical symptoms, mobility, emotional life, and social interaction. Further, these various areas warrant assessment and commensurate intervention over time. For instance, fatigue is a frequent, frustrating, and often disabling symptom in MS that has a major impact on quality of life. Similarly, quality of life in MS is often negatively affected by depression and cognitive dysfunction.

Clinical Pearl
Asking Clients About Their Needs and Desires

Supportive others often feel lost when trying to figure out the "right" thing to say or do to help their loved one. Often, the question "What concerns you the most?" can facilitate a discussion based on the individual's needs and desires. Rather than assuming what the individual could benefit from and then acting on this (potentially well-intended but misguided) assumption, this question allows clients to obtain the support they truly desire.

Given the unpredictable course, many individuals face considerable uncertainty and anxiety, leaving them feeling overwhelmed. As a result, a variety of psychosocial-relevant questions and statements may be posed by individuals living with MS:

- "I feel lost. I am not sure of who I am anymore or what the future holds for me."
- "I am broken."
- "How long will this last?"
- "My emotions now are so raw and hard to control."
- "Should I tell my boss?"
- "I don't think I'll ever find somebody…who would want to sign up for this?"
- "I feel useless."
- "He thinks I'm lazy. He just does not understand what happens to me when fatigue hits."
- "Using the walker feels like I'm just giving up on myself."
- "My attention problems make it difficult to carry on a meaningful conversation."

1.2 Definition

MS is a chronic progressive neurologic disease that impacts the brain and spinal cord (also known as the CNS) as well as other select areas, such as the optic nerves. The CNS conducts electrical and chemical signals throughout the body to allow for thought, emotion, sensory perception, and muscle control. In MS, the flow of information within the brain, and communication between the brain and body, is disrupted.

The precise cause of MS has yet to be established. MS is widely believed to be an immune-mediated disease (NMSS, http://www.nationalmssociety.org/What-is-MS/Definition-of-MS/Immune-mediated-disease). This implies that there is a dysregulation of the normal immune response to some infection or environmental trigger in an individual with genetic vulnerability. The specialized cells and organs that comprise the immune system work in concert to defend the body against attacks by foreign invaders, such as bacteria or viruses. In autoimmune diseases, such as MS, the immune system erroneously identifies self as foreign and assaults select areas of the body that it no longer recognizes. In MS, random attacks of inflammation occur in areas of the white matter and result in significant damage. Within the CNS, white matter acts as

MS is largely thought to be an immune-mediated disease

Table 6
Nervous System Communication Disruption in MS

Motor signals

- Information from the CNS (brain and spinal cord) is transmitted to muscles and other organs through the peripheral nervous system (PNS; the nerves and axons that connect the CNS to muscles, sensory organs, and glands).
- These messages control movement, dexterity, strength, coordination, and other functions of the body.
- Increased muscle tone, resulting in stiffness and spasms, which is referred to as spasticity, is common.
- For example, an individual describes weakness or heaviness in a limb, or a tendency to trip or fall, or drags the affected leg.

Sensory signals

- Sensory organs that provide sensations of vision, hearing, temperature, and touch send messages back to the CNS about the environment.
- For example, an individual expresses concerns about vague and transient symptoms, and describes squeezing, burning, or pressure in a band-like distribution around the chest. Alternatively, the individual may report numbness, prickling, or tingling (also referred to as paresthesias); they may exhibit Lhermitte's sign (i.e., the radiation of tingling or electric-like paresthesias into the limbs or trunk after flexion of the neck).

Integrative signals

- Information is transmitted from nerve to nerve within the nervous system.
- For example, an individual expresses concerns about attention, memory, problem solving, and other cognitive functions.

Note. Adapted from Kalb, Holland, and Giesser (2007)

a relay and coordinates communication between different brain regions. These attacks are commonly referred to as relapses, exacerbations, or flare-ups. As a result of these attacks, nerve impulses slow or stop, and this disruption causes the symptoms experienced by individuals with MS (see Table 6).

The myelin sheath is the protective insulation that surrounds nerve fibers in the white matter of the brain and spinal cord. Myelin facilitates the rapid transmission of electrochemical impulses between the brain, spinal cord, and other body regions (NMSS, http://www.nationalmssociety.org/What-is-MS/Definition-of-MS/Myelin). Myelin is lost in *multiple* areas, leaving scarred or *sclerotic* (hardened) tissue, which gives the disease its name (see Figure 1). The target of destruction includes not only the myelin sheath but also axonal and neuronal degeneration. As such, gray matter can also be impacted early in the disease course. Involvement of gray matter, which implies that there has been destruction of the nerve fibers, has been implicated in irreversible disability (i.e., reduction in function).

The production of lesions and axonal loss results in potential sensory, motor, cognitive, and/or neuropsychiatric difficulties

The collective damage to white and gray matter results in a broad spectrum of clinical signs and symptoms. For instance, symptoms may include sensory problems (e.g., visual disturbances, reduced sensation), motor difficulties (e.g., walking, balance, and coordination problems), cognitive dysfunction (e.g., problems with attention, processing speed, and memory), and changes in

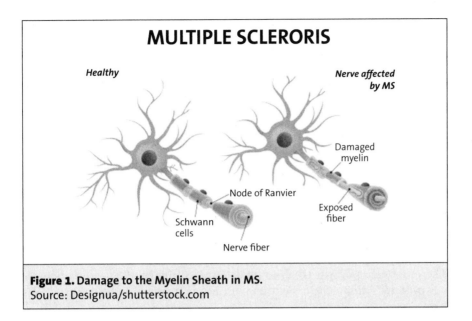

MULTIPLE SCLERORIS

Healthy

Nerve affected
by MS

Damaged
myelin

Node of Ranvier

Exposed
fiber

Schwann
cells

Nerve fiber

Figure 1. Damage to the Myelin Sheath in MS.
Source: Designua/shutterstock.com

mood and behavior. These symptoms may range from mild to severe. Regardless of the level of severity, symptoms can have a significant impact on functioning. Fatigue, for example, is considered by many to be their most disabling symptom. Often individuals describe much angst surrounding the impact of fatigue on their capacity to engage in meaningful activities, such as occupational and home responsibilities as well as hobbies and social events. Likewise, the client's participation in counseling may be challenged whether the disturbance in functioning is isolated or presents in conjunction with other changes. For instance, clients may present with concentration problems that affect discourse during a session, as they lose track of what they wanted to say or have difficulty holding in mind comments made by the therapist. Other clients may grapple with leg weakness and physical pain that makes it difficult to come to therapy to address the onset of emotional dysregulation that has also come about as a symptom of MS.

Particular symptoms also depend on the location of the plaques and can vary greatly. Disease innervating the brain stem, optic nerve, and spinal cord can have more impact on independence. Inflammatory problems of the optic nerve (i.e., optic neuritis) manifest in 55% of persons living with MS. Optic neuritis is often viewed as an early sign of MS, since it presents as the initial symptom in approximately 15% of individuals living with MS. The individual may express concerns about blurred or double vision, color distortion, or even blindness in one eye. Similarly, many describe muscle weakness in their extremities as well as balance and coordination problems at some time point in the disease course.

Someone with MS often faces uncertainty over the duration of MS-related symptoms, which may range from being brief to prolonged. Partial or complete remission of symptoms can occur, particularly in the early stages. Although remission of symptoms is associated with reduced inflammation, progressive structural changes often include volume loss (also known as *atrophy*). The progressive and accumulative nerve damage experienced by individuals living with MS over time is referred to as *neurodegeneration*. The following list illustrates the significant aspects that define the mechanisms of this disease process:

- Inflammatory attacks destroy myelin and oligodendrocytes (the cells that make and maintain myelin).
- Produces damaged areas (lesions or scars) along the nerve.
- Damage and loss of the underlying nerve fiber (axonal damage and atrophy).
- Slows or stops nerve conduction, producing the neurologic signs and symptoms of MS.

1.3   Epidemiology

The exact cause of MS is yet to be determined. Immunologic, environmental, infectious, and genetic contributing factors continue to be explored (see Table 7).

1.3.1   Incidence and Prevalence

The incidence of a disease is the number of new cases occurring in a given period of time

Prevalence refers to the number of people with MS at a particular point in time in a particular place

Some estimates have suggested that there are more than 500,000 people living with MS in the United States and Canada, and more than 2.1 million worldwide (NMSS, 2012).

The prevalence rates for MS vary by continent and geographical latitude (NMSS, http://www.nationalmssociety.org/What-is-MS/Who-Gets-MS). Studies indicate that MS varies greatly in frequency worldwide (Simpson, Blizzard, Otahal, Van der Mei, & Taylor, 2011). Epidemiological statistics on MS have inherent biases, however, which should be kept in mind (see Section 1.3.2 for further detail).

1.3.2   Underdiagnosis of MS

MS remains underdiagnosed, especially among populations of people who do not traditionally participate in biomedical or social science research

As information accumulates, biomedical and psychosocial research findings will uncover the actual incidence and prevalence of the disease, improve the time to an accurate diagnosis, and identify additional treatments that affect the course and severity of the disease.

Inherent Biases and Salient Factors
Epidemiological statistics regarding MS have inherent biases, and, therefore, the estimates of the incidence and prevalence of MS are only approximations.

- There is no single test for MS. The diagnosis can be missed, be delayed, or even be incorrect.
- Data from earlier epidemiological studies may not accurately represent the current MS population because the investigators used different methods for identifying and counting people with MS, as well as different strategies for analyzing their data.

Table 7
Epidemiology of MS

Epidemiological aspects	Details
Age	• MS is the most common neurologic disorder and cause of disability diagnosed in young adults. • MS is typically diagnosed between the ages of 20 and 50 years (NMSS, 2012). • Pediatric MS is diagnosed when MS appears before the age of 16 years (Inaloo & Haghbin, 2013). About 5% of patients present before the age of 16 years but less than 1% before the age of 10 (Gadoth, 2003). • The prevalence of pediatric MS varies by geographic region ranging from 1.35 to 2.5 per 100,000 in the United States to over 248 per 100,000 in western Canada (Renoux et al., 2007).
Gender	• MS is more common in women than men by a ratio of 3.1:2 (NMSS, 2012), with hormones likely to play a determining role in susceptibility.
Ethnicity	• MS occurs in most ethnic and racial groups.
Genetic susceptibility	• Research has suggested that MS develops in individuals who are born with a genetic predisposition that reacts to some environmental agent. Upon exposure to that agent, the autoimmune response is thought to be triggered. • In the general population, the risk of MS is 1/750 (NMSS, 2012). • If one person in a family has MS, their first-degree relatives (e.g., parents, children, and siblings) have a 1–3% chance of getting the disease. • Given that the rate for identical twins both developing MS is significantly lower than 100%, the disease is thought to not be entirely determined by genetics and may be secondary to exposure to something in the environment.
Environmental factors	• The factors within the environment that cause MS to become active have yet to be determined; however, most believe that some unidentified infectious agent, either viral or bacterial, is responsible (NMSS, 2012). • Viruses: Demyelination and inflammation have been shown to result from viruses, suggesting it is possible that a virus or other infectious agent is the trigger in MS. According to the NMSS, more than a dozen viruses and bacteria – including measles, canine distemper, human herpes virus 6, Epstein–Barr, and *Chlamydophila pneumoniae* – have been or are being investigated to determine involvement in the development of MS, but none have been definitively proven to trigger MS (Serafini et al., 2007).
Potential modifiable risk factors	• Research is accumulating evidence regarding potential risk factors, including obesity, tobacco use, and vitamin D levels.

- Longitudinal data can be skewed toward individuals who had more progressive symptoms. Prior to the arrival of disease modifiers, people who had more mild symptoms or whose health was stable and were managing well were usually not included in the studies.
- Diagnostic procedures are complicated and expensive, making them unavailable to people with poor or no health coverage, people in rural or impoverished areas, and people whose language or level of education prevented them from both advocating for appropriate referrals and testing and navigating the complicated and confusing diagnostic process.
- MS is not a "reportable" disease, which means that the government does not require physicians to inform any central database when they make the diagnosis. Without this kind of centralized reporting system, there is no easy way to accurately count people with MS.

1.3.3   Psychiatric Diagnoses in MS

Mood Disorders

Based on data collected largely from individuals attending MS clinics, depression has been reported as the most common psychiatric disorder in this population (Minden & Schiffer, 1990), with the lifetime prevalence of major depressive disorder in MS estimated to be around 50%. This estimate is 3 times that of the general population. Moreover, a quarter of MS patients suffer from suicidal ideation, and the risk of suicide is 5–10 times higher than in the general population (Feinstein, 2002).

Clients may also report difficulty regulating their emotions. Although equivocal, the prevalence of bipolar disorders in MS has been estimated to be twice that in the general population (Schiffer, Wineman, & Weitkamp, 1986). Pseudobulbar affect syndrome, which reflects incongruent affect characterized by sudden uncontrollable outbursts of laughter or crying, has been reported in approximately 10% of individuals with MS (Ghaffar & Feinstein, 2007). Pseudobulbar affect has been associated with more extensive disease and longer duration of MS, as well as greater rates of cognitive dysfunction and disability.

Anxiety

Estimates of the prevalence of anxiety in MS are extremely variable, ranging from 19% to 90%. Among those individuals who are newly diagnosed, higher rates of anxiety have been found (34%), documenting that this is an anxiety-provoking time for these individuals. According to Korostil and Feinstein (2007), the prevalence of specific diagnoses vary: Examples include generalized anxiety disorder (18.6%), panic disorder (10%), obsessive-compulsive disorder (8.6%), and social anxiety disorder (7.8%). Heightened anxiety has also been shown in partners of persons living with MS (40%; Janssens et al., 2003).

Psychosis

Prevalence rates of psychosis are 2–3% among persons living with MS compared with 0.5–1% in the general population. In contrast to schizophrenia, individuals with MS tend to rarely exhibit negative symptoms, but instead tend to experience complex delusions. Demyelinating lesion location has been associated with psychosis, such as reports of high bilateral lesion load in the medial temporal regions (Feinstein, du Boulay, & Ron, 1992). Psychosis may result from the medication effects associated with drugs such as steroids and interferons.

Cognitive Impairment

Previously, it was believed that cognitive impairment only occurred rarely and in severe cases of MS, even though cognitive impairment has been documented since the earliest clinical descriptions of MS. At present, cognitive deficits are recognized as a prevalent and disabling consequence of MS. According to Julian (2011), prevalence rates of cognitive decline fall in the range of 40–65% of persons with MS, while rates obtained from clinical settings range from 53% to 65% and are slightly lower in community studies, at about 45%. Cognitive deficits are found in approximately one third of children with MS (Weisbrot et al., 2014).

1.4   Course and Prognosis

1.4.1   Course

The clinical presentation and course of MS is highly variable. Although the unpredictable nature of the disease process is a hallmark feature, descriptions of the course such as intermittent, episodic, chronic, and progressive may be used to characterize this neurological disease.

> The course of MS is heterogeneous, given the variability of symptoms and unpredictable onset of changes

Over the course of the disease, signs and symptoms can be quite heterogeneous. Individuals with MS may express uncertainty regarding whether or not a symptom is related to MS or results from some other contributing factor. A typical example of this occurs when an individual notes that fatigue is disabling and interferes with the quality of their work and home life, yet does not know if fatigue is due to MS, life stressors, medication effects, sleep fragmentation, or depression. Still, as a nonspecific symptom, fatigue can simultaneously be due to more than one condition within the same individual (e.g., MS and depression). Through comprehensive assessment and monitoring, the main contributing factors to be addressed in treatment can be identified.

The course of MS is marked by symptoms that vary from mild to disabling, with acute exacerbations that are not anticipated. During the early course of the disease, exacerbations consist of subacute neurological symptoms that worsen over days to a few weeks, with spontaneous and complete recovery often described. Despite this, residual deficits may continue to exist. Moreover, the symptoms and signs can also contribute to the steady progression of the disease (Milo & Miller, 2014).

Clinical Pearl
Understanding the Course and Prognosis of MS

Integration of the diagnosis into the individual's sense of self and daily living, as well as plans for the future often depend on understanding the course and prognosis.

- Some MS course subtypes can be characterized by an abrupt onset that adversely impacts functioning, with a course that comes and goes in transient episodes. This course can be described as unpredictable flare-ups interspersed with periods of stability. The individual living with MS may initially experience shock, fear, disbelief, and confusion. The patient's time and energies are consumed by the symptom(s) and corresponding treatment. Physical and/or cognitive difficulties can challenge autonomy, particularly during the acute phase. The experience may induce exhaustion in supportive others who provide primary assistance (e.g., coordinating urgent medical visits, addressing the increased need for practical and emotional support), but eventually their focus returns to getting on with regular life. The individual and/or family may notice a preoccupation with anticipatory grief and distress about the unpredictable nature of the course and prognosis.

- Individuals and supportive others can adjust to living with MS in a variety of ways. Areas to assess may include:
  - How flexible or rigid is the individual/family in adjusting to change?
  - Are they innovative about changing established rules and adjusting cultural values/mores, or are they reticent to make changes in social roles?
  - Do they take on a proactive, problem-solving focus in their strategies to address weaknesses?
  - Do they tend to stay in "crisis mode," or do they plan ahead?
  - How cohesive and engaged are they in understanding MS (as a family unit, in their intimate relationship or friendship), making treatment-related decisions as a couple/family, and accessing resources (e.g., medical, rehabilitative, supportive, legal, and financial) together?
  - How well do they address salient issues, such as independence and intimacy?

Although the established clinical phenotypes associated with different disease courses are listed below, refined descriptors that include consideration of disease activity (based upon clinical relapse rate and imaging findings) are being proposed by MS specialists and researchers (Lublin et al., 2014).

Relapsing–Remitting MS (RRMS)

MS is a disorder where "one size" will not fit all – MS is clinically divided into relapsing and progressive subtypes

RRMS is characterized by clearly defined acute attacks with full recovery or with residual deficit upon recovery (NMSS, http://www.nationalmssociety.org/What-is-MS/Types-of-MS/Relapsing-remitting-MS). The periods between disease relapses are characterized by a lack of disease progression. Approximately 85% of people are diagnosed initially with RRMS (Lublin & Reingold, 1996).

Clinically Isolated Syndrome (CIS)

The course of MS is difficult to predict, especially at onset

A temporary diagnosis of clinically isolated syndrome (CIS) may initially be given if insufficient brain MRI evidence is present when a person with MS is first evaluated. Such a label implies increased risk for future confirmed MS, given the need for subsequent evidence of further clinical relapses or new MRI lesions. More than two thirds of individuals with CIS who also have abnormal MRI findings convert to a diagnosis of MS (Tintoré et al., 2006).

Secondary Progressive MS (SPMS)

Following an initial relapsing–remitting course, the disease transitions in many people to a steadily progressive form with increased loss of function, characterized by nerve damage or loss. Individuals may or may not continue to experience relapses caused by inflammation. Of the 85% who start with RRMS, more than 50% will develop SPMS within 10 years and 90% within 25 years.

Primary Progressive MS (PPMS)

A minority of patients avoid the relapsing–remitting disease phase, but develop a primary progressive course from the onset (Leary, 2007; Lublin & Reingold, 1996); approximately 10% of MS patients have PPMS. Typically, the onset of PPMS occurs in mid-life, in the 40s or 50s, and is characterized by disease progression from onset, without distinct relapses. However, others have noted that the PPMS course may include occasional plateaus and temporary minor improvements (Milo & Miller, 2014). PPMS is associated with relatively less evidence of inflammatory activity (subsequent clinical relapses and MRI lesions) than RRMS, and likely represents a neurodegenerative process (Miller et al., 2007).

Progressive Relapsing MS (PRMS)

PRMS is marked by progressive disease from onset, with occasional acute relapses and continuing disease progression. The physician may initially diagnose the person as having PPMS and then modify the diagnosis when the first relapse occurs (NMSS, http://www.nationalmssociety.org/What-is-MS/Types-of-MS/Progressive-relapsing-MS/Diagnosing-Progressive-Relapsing-MS). PRMS is the least common presentation, and approximately 5% of people appear to have PRMS at diagnosis.

RRMS is the most often occurring course, and PRMS is the least common

Pediatric Onset

Pediatric MS is defined as the appearance of MS before the age of 16 years. Acute exacerbations occur more frequently in pediatric patients than in adult patients, and exacerbations are 3 times more frequent in pediatric patients than in adult-onset patients (Yeh & Weinstock-Guttman, 2012). Clinical features of pediatric and adult MS are similar. Despite this, optic neuritis, isolated brain stem syndrome, and symptoms of encephalopathy like headache, vomiting, seizure, and/or altered consciousness are more common in children (Renoux et al., 2007). Approximately 97–99% of children with MS experience RRMS, whereas PPMS is rare in children (Inaloo & Haghbin, 2013).

1.4.2   Prognosis

A rare variant of MS, known as *malignant MS*, causes a rapid deterioration resulting in significant disability or even death shortly after disease onset. A benign course that reflects minimal disease activity has been described in approximately 10–15% of individuals living with MS (Lublin & Reingold,

Life expectancy is mildly affected in MS

1996; Mohr & Cox, 2001). However, continuous pathological activity is associated with disease progression and accumulation of disability over time (Milo & Miller, 2014). Relapse frequency actually tends to diminish over time and with increasing age in MS patients.

Specific variables predict long-term prognosis. For example, male gender is associated with a less favorable outcome (Damasceno, Von Glehn, Brandão, Damasceno, & Cendes, 2013). By contrast, younger age at onset has been proposed as a positive prognostic indicator.

Pregnancy is an important issue for a large proportion of women with MS. The 3-month period after giving birth has been identified as a high-risk period for MS attacks, with approximately 30% of untreated individuals experiencing a relapse (Coyle et al., 2014). The relapse rate reportedly decreases in the last trimester of pregnancy. Recent studies suggest the long-term prognosis may be more favorable in relapsing MS when individuals experience one or more pregnancies. Of note, individuals with MS show no increased risk for miscarriage.

1.4.3   Treatment Effects on Course and Prognosis

The interaction between treatment and course will influence prognostic outcomes

At present, there is no cure for MS. During acute relapses, steroids may be prescribed, as they have been shown to limit the duration and severity of attacks for some individuals. In RRMS, residual effects of clinical relapses often result in accumulating neurological impairment (Lublin, Baier, & Cutter, 2003). Distinguishing RRMS from PPMS is crucial because all available MS disease-modifying treatments (DMTs) are efficacious for reducing attacks in relapsing MS, but have not yet been proven to affect PPMS (Wingerchuk & Carter, 2014). Medications are used to modify the disease course, treat relapses, and manage symptoms, with rehabilitation employed to reduce impairment and improve activity and participation. In RRMS, DMTs decrease the development of new cortical lesions and reduce the progression of cortical atrophy compared with untreated individuals (Calabrese et al., 2012). Naturally occurring antiviral proteins known as interferons have been shown to reduce the number of exacerbations and to slow progression of physical disability. Immunosuppressive agents may also influence the course of the disease.

1.4.4   Course and Prognosis of MS Signs and Symptoms

Course and Prognosis of Psychiatric Diagnoses in MS

Depressive symptoms are often prolonged in patients with MS. Longitudinal data collected from individuals with MS and comorbid depressive symptoms showed that 10-year follow-up depression scores were not significantly different from baseline (Koch, Uyttenboogaart, Van Harten, Heerings, & De Keyser, 2008). Overall, depression is not clearly associated with disability scores or disease course (with the majority of regression models finding no significant associations). These findings argue against interpreting prolonged depression as a reaction to worsening disability. Similarly, interferon treatment for MS was initially associated with depression, but this has not been substantiated by the bulk of subsequent studies. Rather, neuroimaging studies on the chronicity of depression in MS support an organic etiology; MRI lesion load and brain atrophy, particularly in the frontal and temporal lobes, have been associated with the presence and severity of depression in MS. The long-term prognosis of depression in MS appears to more closely resemble criteria for persistent depressive disorder (Koch et al., 2014).

Similarly, anxiety is related with disease activity, but not with disease duration or severity (Noy et al., 1995). General and MS-specific worry (e.g., obtaining medication, financial problems related to having MS, being a "burden" to family) are elevated and common in people living with MS. Healthcare worry is related to greater depressive symptoms, anxiety, fatigue, sleep disturbance, and pain interference, as well as worse social function and perceived cognitive dysfunction (Jones & Amtmann, 2014). Further, the disease course and prognosis are affected, as MS-specific worries have been shown to be related to worse health.

Course and Prognosis of Cognitive Impairment in MS

Cognitive deficits are now recognized as one of the leading causes of disability among individuals living with MS. While not all individuals experience cognitive problems, such difficulties can occur across all stages of the illness. In later disease stages, cognitive dysfunction becomes both more prevalent and more severe.

In MS, variables that may affect cognitive functioning include depression, disease type, and disability status (Johnson, 2007). Yet cognitive deficits are not closely correlated with physical impairment. Despite this, cognitive dysfunction is associated with lesion burden and diffuse disease, as well as subcortical atrophy and ventricle enlargement (Johnson, 2007).

Individuals with progressive types of MS usually demonstrate more marked cognitive impairment. Similarly, the disease course may influence the type of cognitive deficits exhibited (Gaudino, Chiaravalloti, DeLuca, & Diamond, 2001). Although not fully substantiated, several studies have demonstrated less severe cognitive and functional deficits in individuals diagnosed with RRMS compared with those with progressive forms of MS (i.e., primary progressive and secondary progressive), particularly with regard to verbal learning and memory. In addition, the interplay between cognition and psychiatric symptoms is also relevant to prognosis. For instance, cognitive decline over a 1-year period was revealed in longitudinal studies that examined individuals with MS who had demonstrated negative affect at baseline (Christodoulou et al., 2009).

Course and Prognosis of Cognitive and Psychiatric Disorders in Pediatric MS

Cognitive and psychiatric symptoms have been reported and tend to occur relatively early in the first 1–2 years of the illness in pediatric populations. However, longitudinal studies are needed to assess the long-term risk and consequence of these symptoms. Immunomodulating treatments, such as interferon beta drugs (interferon beta-1a and 1b) and glatiramer acetate, are used to prevent relapses or progression of MS. In adults, these interventions have been shown to reduce the recurrence rate of MS by 30%; however, no randomized controlled trials have been conducted to study the effect of these treatments on MS in children (Inaloo & Haghbin, 2013). These findings underscore the importance of the development of early interventions (Yeh & Weinstock-Guttman, 2012).

1.5   Differential Diagnosis

1.5.1   Symptoms of MS Versus Other Etiologies

As noted by Minden and colleagues (2014), mood (persistent inner emotional states) and disturbances of affect (changing external expression of emotions) are affected by MS.

MS-Related Symptoms Versus Mood Disorders

Fatigue may be attributed to a comorbid depressive disorder, although this is not always applicable. Indeed, psychological well-being is impacted by an individual's reduced control over fatigue and other MS-related problems. Likewise, symptoms such as changes in sleep, appetite, or libido may be secondary to a comorbid medical condition, MS, medication effects, or psychiatric disorders. Although rare, individuals with MS can exhibit pathological laughter or crying related to brain areas impacted by MS. The syndrome of emotional lability (pseudobulbar affect) is sometimes misinterpreted as bipolar disorder. Lastly, treatment can impact mood. For instance, short-term corticosteroid therapy, which may be used to treat acute phases of MS relapses, can produce mood disorder, euphoria, and hypomania, as well as depressive symptoms subsequent to long-term corticosteroid therapy.

MS-Related Symptoms Versus Psychosis

Psychosis can be associated with specific lesion location (i.e., a higher lesion load in the medial temporal lobe regions bilaterally). In addition, all clinicians should evaluate the potential psychosis-inducing effects of medications such as steroids and interferons.

Clinical Pearl
Teasing Apart Symptoms Related to MS or Other Conditions

Consulting with other specialists can help tease apart whether a symptom is MS-related or due to another condition (e.g., a comorbid medical problem, medication effect, or a psychiatric issue). Mental health professionals should consult with a neurologist or other professionals for fully informed assessment and treatment planning. For instance, significantly reduced energy may be secondary to depression, obstructive sleep apnea, medication side effects, or MS-type fatigue.

- An onset or worsening of symptoms does not necessarily translate to disease progression. That is, an attack may actually be a "pseudoexacerbation" and result from an infection (e.g., urinary tract infection), exhaustion, psychosocial difficulties, or psychiatric disorder(s).

- Assuming that the disease process is "progressing" may be erroneous, as other culprits may include decreased exercise, insufficient access to resources/treatment or modifications, and/or other physical or psychological problems.

1.5.2   Psychiatric Diagnoses

Somatic Symptom Disorders

MS can manifest in the absence of objective data found in neurological examinations, leading the diagnosis to be confused with a psychiatric disorder such as a somatic symptom disorder. The DSM-5 (American Psychiatric Association, 2013) has refocused the classification of somatic symptom disorders, and simply having an unexplained symptom is not a sufficient cause for establishing a psychiatric diagnosis. Alternatively, the presence of a well-documented medical symptom does not exclude the possibility of a dysfunctional psychological reaction that would be an appropriate focus for treatment. Functional neurological symptoms refer to neurological symptoms that are not explained by disease, and approximately one third of neurology outpatients have symptoms that neurologists rate as only "somewhat" or "not at all" explained by disease (Stone, Reuber, & Carson, 2013). Examples of diagnostic-related issues include: (1) a diagnostic error: "Patient presented with symptoms that were plausibly all due to MS but was diagnosed with functional symptoms. The diagnosis of MS had not been considered and was unexpected at follow-up"; or (2) a differential diagnostic change: "Patient presented with multiple symptoms. Doctor suggested chronic fatigue syndrome as most likely but considered MS as a possible diagnosis. Appropriate investigations and follow-up confirmed MS."

Reactive Versus Organic Mood Disturbance

Mood disturbances in MS (e.g., anxiety, depression) may be reactive in nature, given that the individual often faces adjustments to physical health, well-being, lifestyle, social roles, and mental health. Indeed, lower levels of depression are associated with active problem solving, coping strategies, and cognitive reframing but not escape–avoidance strategies (Mohr et al., 1997). Alternatively, an organic basis (e.g., particular brain regions impacted by MS, neurophysiologic changes, medication effects) may explain mood and affective disturbances in MS. Depression, for example, may occur in response to immunological and inflammatory changes and structural changes, such as atrophy and brain lesions (Marrie et al., 2015). Still, the confluence of both organic and reactive contributors may be present.

1.5.3   Neuropsychological Diagnosis

In addition to physical signs and symptoms, MS may affect neuropsychological functioning, influencing mood, behavior, and cognition. However, neuropsychological symptoms can occur in the absence of any physical problems or they can co-occur with sensory or motoric changes. If left unidentified and untreated, neuropsychological issues can adversely affect quality of life (Pepping & Ehde, 2005). Clients can express frustration, self-doubt, helplessness, and apprehension regarding the impact of their cognitive problems, and independence can be compromised by cognitive difficulties. For some individuals, even subtle cognitive problems or neurobehavioral symptoms can challenge adjustment, and these clients are more apt to experience heightened

Even subtle cognitive or neurobehavioral problems can challenge adjustment

Discussion about cognitive functioning should be facilitated by mental health providers throughout treatment

distress related to cognitive declines that impact work and home demands. Individuals who experience cognitive dysfunction are often at risk of loss of employment. Moderate to severe cognitive dysfunction is associated with declines in performing activities of daily living (e.g., driving, financial management, household chores). Significant cognitive difficulties often require additional assistance from supportive others and/or professionals. The neuropsychological evaluation serves as the framework that allows for a plan tailored to an individual and his or her support network.

Clinical Pearl
Neuropsychological Consultation

Consider a referral for neuropsychological evaluation when you encounter any of the following scenarios:

- The client passes a brief cognitive screen administered by a healthcare professional but continues to express concern about neuropsychological declines and functional problems; request an objective assessment of the nature and extent of neuropsychological dysfunction using more sensitive and specific standardized measures.

- The client is trying to decide whether or not to obtain disability benefits or continue working. If the quality of their job performance is compromised, clients often wish to learn strategies to address their employers' concerns as well as identify workplace modifications and accommodations that they may be legally eligible to receive.

- Supportive others, colleagues, or employers have expressed concerns to the individual or directly to the mental health professional about the individual's cognitive and/or neurobehavioral functioning, but the client has limited awareness of these problems.

- The mental health professional suspects that cognitive and/or neurobehavioral problems are interfering with treatment progress and would like objective data as well as professional consultation to assess what may prove useful to facilitate the goals of intervention.

- When trying to determine how role-reactive emotional issues may be affecting the person's cognitive presentation (i.e., the influence of psychiatric overlay on cognitive performance).

- When determining issues of practical importance, such as living alone, relocating to an assisted living or a skilled nursing facility, driving, or other capacity-related issues (e.g., financial and/or healthcare management).

- To provide assessment and consultation regarding behavioral management and environmental modifications for individuals who demonstrate neuropsychiatric symptoms (e.g., reduced insight, impulsivity, apathy, mood lability, diminished initiation, anger control problems) that can cause significant functional impairment and distress for the client and/or their support network.

The cognitive deficits that an individual with MS may encounter can either reflect a magnification of preexisting weaknesses or a marked change in ability. For instance, someone who may have always struggled with expressing his or her thoughts in a straightforward manner may now report that others have become irritated because he or she is too disorganized and tangential during conversations. Moreover, cognitive changes often result in marked distress for the individual. Yet, other individuals may have always performed well in an environment where great demands can be placed upon multitasking and rapid responding (e.g., nurse, chef), but now they struggle to switch their attention or get stuck in the details while working on a project.

Cognitive difficulties may range from subtle to significant

Cognitive problems are often misattributed. For instance, others may misidentify slowed processing speed or inattention as disinterest, laziness, or lack of effort. Family members, friends, and employers may assume that the client is manipulating a situation, shows diminished affection, lacks motivation, or is simply irresponsible. This results in faulty attribution for the actual cognitive weakness or neurobehavioral symptom that has yet to be accurately identified. Clients can question whether their cognitive problems are due to other diagnoses, such as Alzheimer's disease or attention deficit disorder, given the limited information that they are provided with on the potential neuropsychological manifestations of MS. When cognitive disruptions occur but are not properly identified, a person with MS may feel guilty, anxious, and overwhelmed. Clients may show a tendency toward self-doubt and isolation as a result, and important others can provide insufficient support. Additionally, neuropsychiatric symptoms, dementia, and cognitive dysfunction in individuals living with MS can be associated with distress and negative feelings in caregivers.

Cognitive difficulties are often mislabeled as "laziness," disinterest, or part of a mood disorder

---

Clinical Pearl
Clearing Up Myths About Cognitive Dysfunction in MS

- Cognitive dysfunction in MS was initially thought to be present only in those individuals with severe and obvious physical difficulties. We now know that cognitive deficits may appear at any point of the disease process and are not associated with level of physical disability (NMSS, http://www. nationalmsso-ciety.org/Symptoms-Diagnosis/MS-Symptoms/Cognitive-Changes).

- The clinical presentation of cognitive impairment in MS is variable. Cognitive weaknesses may range from mild or subtle difficulties to marked impairment, but it is very rare for clients to meet DSM-5 criteria for dementia. Most individuals who seek neuropsychological evaluation or cognitive rehabilitation present with mild cognitive concerns.

- Someone can develop a specific cognitive deficit that is related to the appearance of a new lesion on MRI, although this is rare. A more frequent presentation involves what are referred to as clinically silent attacks in which white matter damage accumulates over time, contributing to cognitive dysfunction.

- Cognitive compensatory strategies, environmental modifications, and participation in rehabilitation (e.g., speech therapy, occupational therapy) can be effective ways to manage cognitive symptoms that arise in MS.

- The mental health professional plays a key role in encouraging individuals living with MS to seek education about cognitive and emotional problems related to MS, types of compensatory strategies, and remaining open to building connections with helpful resources.

Remaining flexible is important; a strategy that worked today may be of little value tomorrow

1.5.4   Types of Cognitive Dysfunction in MS

Information Processing Speed

The most frequently observed impairment observed in MS appears to be reduced information processing speed. Processing speed refers to the rapidity with which a person is able to perform a mental activity. This includes the speed with which one can process auditory or visual material/information, such as processing information during a conversation or while reading.

Typical Problems
- Day-to-day tasks are more time-consuming.
- Losing track of time or not allotting enough time for an activity or project.
- Difficulty keeping up with the flow of conversation.
- Feeling "drained" from increased effort to process information.
- Others misinterpreting slowed processing speed for disinterest.

Influencing Factors
- A variety of medications, including anticonvulsants, can slow information processing.
- The efficiency of the frontal lobes in organizing and directing information flow; impaired self-regulation (or executive dysfunction) can result in slowed processing because of weak control over attention, organization, memory, and other cognitive processes.
- Slow processing can be a consequence of depression or anxiety, or simply a focus on unrelated issues as a result of emotional struggles.

Attention, Concentration, Working Memory

Individuals living with MS often have trouble with attention, and they frequently encounter problems with vigilance. Attentional problems are likely to increase over time when MS clients are required to persist on a demanding task. Cognitive fatigue contributes to diminished mental stamina and vigilance over longer periods. Clients often benefit when they reduce their stress level related to the task, take breaks, and eliminate distractions. Also, working memory problems are common. Working memory refers to the capacity to hold information in mind for further mental manipulation, learning, and processing. While basic attention is preserved, problems in attention are more likely to be encountered as information becomes more detailed and complex. The variability of attention control issues is described in the following list:

a. Selective attention (focus)
- The ability to maintain concentration with competing distractions.
- Example: Attending to one conversation at a dinner table while other conversations are also taking place.

b. Alternating/shifting attention (flexibility)
- The ability to alternate or shift attention between two or more tasks.
- Examples: Working in an office answering phones, checking e-mail, and shifting between typing and responding to inquiries. Making dinner and stopping to put laundry in the dryer.

c. Sustained attention (concentration; vigilance; working memory)
- The ability to maintain concentration over a period of time.
- Example: Reading for 30 min.

d. Divided attention (multitasking)
- The ability to respond simultaneously to multiple tasks or demands.
- Example: Driving a car and listening to the radio or carrying on a conversation.

Typical Problems
- Difficulty sustaining mental effort on a task (i.e., vigilance).
- Mind wanders onto other issues.
- Becoming flustered or feeling frustrated after losing train of thought.
- Feeling overwhelmed on tasks that require sustained attention.
- Problems holding information in mind (i.e., working memory).
- Difficulty following multiple-step instructions.
- "Shutting down" or avoiding crowds or environments that trigger feeling overwhelmed and/or over stimulated; having difficulty focusing because of over-sensitivity to sights, sounds, movement.

Influencing Factors
- MS-related neurophysiologic changes.
- Medication effects.
- Physical status: fatigue, pain, hunger, bladder/bowel issues.
- Emotions.
- Interest level.
- Demands (competing interpersonal or attentional demands; multiple requests; overstimulation from the environment from various sensory inputs).

Verbal and Visual Learning and Memory

Initially, researchers conceptualized memory dysfunction in MS to be solely indicative of a retrieval deficit (i.e., a client has poor free recall but benefits from prompts, cues, and recognition formats). For instance, a client may have difficulty recalling the content of a conversation but his capacity to provide information about it can improve when he is given some hints or short reminders about key topics discussed. While a pattern of retrieval problems can exist, additional research has revealed that the initial amount of new information learned or acquired is adversely impacted. The acquisition phase of new learning is the initial stage of memory and can be compromised by weaknesses in processing speed and attention.

Typical Problems
- Difficulty recalling information from conversations.
- Misplacing objects.
- Problems recalling how to get places (particularly when using unfamiliar routes).

Influencing Factors
- MS-related neurophysiologic changes.
- Attention.
- Processing speed.
- Physical status: fatigue, pain, hunger, bladder/bowel issues.
- Emotions.
- Importance or salience of the information.

Executive Functions

Executive functions are those abilities that allow us to engage in purposeful, goal-directed behavior. They involve skills necessary for planning and organization, volition, purposeful action, and effective performance. From a neuropsychological perspective, executive functioning can reflect the capacity to maintain appropriate control over one's thoughts, behaviors, and emotions (i.e., regulation) and the ability to manage one's attention and problem solving (i.e., metacognition).

Typical Problems
- Difficulty with cognitive flexibility (a tendency to show rigid thinking or not consider alternatives).
- Disinhibition (impulsive responding).
- Poor abstraction, reasoning, planning, problem solving, organization, prioritizing, initiation, and self-monitoring of behavior.
- Limited use of feedback to guide performance.

Influencing Factors
- MS-related neurophysiologic changes, particularly implicating frontal systems functioning.

Visuospatial Perception

Visual perception can be affected by MS. Visual problems, such as residual effects of optic neuritis, can hamper visuospatial skills, although the types of problems described often have to do with the areas of the brain that are responsible for understanding and perceiving visual information.

Typical Problems
- Poor sense of direction or disorientation in space.

Influencing Factors
- MS-related neurophysiologic changes, particularly those that involve the visual cortex.

Language

While language abilities largely remain unchanged, a common concern involves word finding, and clients can lose confidence in their capacity to hold meaningful conversations. They can become flustered and frustrated by tip-of-the-tongue searches for words. A reciprocal relationship often evolves, as word-finding disturbance is exacerbated by emotional upset and vice versa. Likewise, others can lose patience or have difficulty following the clients' line of thought when this problem occurs.

Typical Problems
- Difficulty thinking of the word a client wishes to use.
- Substituting words (sometimes semantically similar, while at others times very different).
- Speaking hesitantly, with great pauses as the client searches for a word.

Influencing Factors
- MS-related neurophysiologic changes.
- Fatigue.
- Weaknesses in attention, processing speed, memory retrieval.
- Emotion.

1.5.5 Neuropsychological Evaluation

A neuropsychological evaluation typically consists of a clinical interview, collateral interview(s), and the administration of standardized measures of cognition, mood, and adaptive functioning. A neuropsychological evaluation can identify cognitive strengths and weaknesses, as well as determine the extent to which the individual's concerns or the concerns of others are attributed to MS and/or other confounding factors (e.g., fatigue, depression, medication effects). The findings of the evaluation can guide treatment planning and help clients understand their difficulties. As Pepping and Ehde (2005) note:

> Informed and compassionate discussion and support from an experienced provider who can understand and describe the person's range of abilities and their key vulnerabilities can provide clarity, a plan for improvement, and a sense of hope that something practical can be done to improve function. (p. 411)

Because the results of the evaluation can be affected by specific MS-related issues (e.g., fatigue, sensory problems, motoric challenges, pain, etc.), we recommend that the referring clinician consult with a neuropsychologist who is experienced in working with clients living with MS.

Patients are often apprehensive about disclosure of neuropsychological evaluation results to others such as family, friends, coworkers, and employers. The neuropsychologist can assist the individual with problem solving about what specific information may be helpful to disclose, to whom the information should be given, and when that information should be shared, as well as provide potentially helpful legal resources and avenues for emotional support when communicating one's weaknesses to others.

1.6   Comorbidities

1.6.1   Medical and Biobehavioral Comorbidities in MS

Sleep Disturbance in MS

Sleep disturbances have been shown to be more prevalent among individuals with MS in contrast to the general population, with prevalence estimates that range from 25% to 54% (Caminero & Bartolomé, 2011; see Table 8). Insomnia, for instance, has been shown to have a prevalence rate higher than 40% compared with 10–15% in the general population. Insomnia can be secondary to spasticity, pain, sexual dysfunction, or bladder issues, and awakening too early in the morning is the most common symptom (58%). As noted by Caminero and Bartolomé (2011), the relationship between psychiatric disorders and sleep disturbances is bidirectional (i.e., insomnia causes depression and anxiety, and vice versa).

Table 8
Sleep Disturbance Secondary to Medications Often Used in MS

Medication (indication)	Sleep disturbance
Baclofen (spasticity)	Sedation
Tizanidine (spasticity)	Daytime sleepiness
Clonazepam (spasticity, tremor)	Sleepiness
Amantadine (chronic fatigue syndrome)	Insomnia
SSRI (chronic fatigue syndrome, anxiety–depression)	Insomnia, sedation
Modafinil (chronic fatigue syndrome)	Insomnia
Gabapentin (neuropathic pain)	Hypersomnia
Carbamazepine (paroxysmal phenomena)	Sedation
Oxybutynin (neurogenic bladder)	Sedation
Interferon beta (disease course modifier)	Insomnia, hypersomnia
Methylprednisolone (anti-inflammatory)	Insomnia

Note. Adapted from A. Caminero and M. Bartolomé (2011)

Stress and MS

Many people living with MS report that stress triggers exacerbations

Dr. Hans Selye first brought the term *stress* into popular culture in the 1950s, based on his studies of the response of animals when injured or placed in extreme conditions. He later coined the term *stressor* to describe the stimulus or event that produced the stress response (Kabat-Zinn, 1990). Put simply, stress is the collection of physiological and psychological changes that occur in response to a psychological or physical stressor.

Chronic psychological stress is associated with the body losing its ability to regulate the inflammatory response (Cohen et al., 2012). In response to psychological stressors, an inflammatory process may occur after release of neuropeptides, or other inflammatory mediators, from sensory nerves and the activation of mast cells or other inflammatory cells (Black, 2002). This is due in part to the flight–fight response of the autonomic nervous system. When there is a stressor the autonomic nervous system prepares the body to either fight the aggressor or flee, initiating a physiological stress response (Porges, 2001). Most stress management techniques involve either preventing or ameliorating this stress response.

While once the relationship between stress and MS was only supported by anecdotal information, a meta-analysis of research on stress and MS documented a relationship between stress and clinical exacerbation (Mohr et al., 2004). More recently, research has supported a connection between stress and the development of new brain lesions. However, Mohr and colleagues (2012) point out that the relationships are not always consistent either within patients or across patients. Mohr et al. (2012) reviewed findings that suggest that psychological, social, and biological factors may be involved in this relationship and argued that a purely causal relationship, in which stressful events alone trigger exacerbation, was unlikely. However, Mohr (2007) found data to suggest that more effective coping strategies may influence the relationship between stress and MS inflammation.

Living with MS often amplifies the more common stressors of relationships, family, work, or money, and it can result in additional stressors as well. These include the daily and long-term unpredictability of the disease, managing medical appointments and medications, adjusting to increasing or fluctuating disability, and navigating daily life tasks with multiple MS symptoms.

Someone living with this disease confronts a double bind: MS is a stressor and stress can increase MS symptoms. Therefore, people living with MS carry the burden of trying to avoid or minimize stress while still trying to live a full life that will inevitably include stress. Dr. Rosalind Kalb of the NMSS states: "People can be so worried about anything making their disease worse that it becomes another stress in and of itself" (http://multiplesclerosis.net).

Pain in MS

Until quite recently, pain was not recognized as a symptom frequently associated with MS. However, research documents that as many as 65% of people with MS report living with pain or discomfort (Kerns, Kassirer, & Otis, 2002). Pain may be caused directly by the disease acting on the nervous system or indirectly through a functional impairment. Further, efforts to medically manage MS may inadvertently exacerbate pain and pain-related disability. Pain can occur with any form of MS and is sometimes reported as being the most difficult symptom for people to manage (Kerns, Kassirer, et al., 2002). Kerns and colleagues report that unresolved pain, associated disability, and affective distress are common in MS.

The psychological effects of pain and its management will often be the focus of psychotherapy

Classification

MS-related pain can be classified by its *origin* (nociceptive or neurogenic) or its *duration* (acute, chronic, or episodic).

Origin and Duration

Nociceptive pain, caused by tissue damage and/or inflammation, is common in the general population, while *neurogenic pain* results from a neurological disorder or spinal cord injury. People with MS may experience both types of pain for any duration (Kerns, Kassirer et al., 2002). Similar to other MS symptoms, pain can be episodic, further complicating management.

Nociceptive Pain
- Coordination difficulties, numbness, and misinterpretation of temperature can result in injury-related pain. Immobility, present with increased disability, can lead to inflammation-based pain.
- Musculoskeletal pain; sprains, strains, pulls, and muscle overuse can develop from falls, gait imbalance, misuse of a mobility aid, or overcompensation.

Table 9
Nervous System Communication Disruption in MS

Name/Subcategory	Symptoms	Duration
Allodynia	Painful sensation in response to innocuous stimulus such as a light touch, bed sheets, or clothes	Episodic, chronic
Dysesthesias	Burning, aching, itching, girdling, or squeezing around the body triggered by a light touch or nothing at all	Episodic, acute, chronic
MS hug: a type of dysesthesia	Felt on torso, encircling the body; sharp or dull, burning or tickling, tingling, crushing or constricting	Chronic, episodic
Paresthesia: similar to dysesthesia	Pins and needles, tingling, buzzing, or vibrating; mild to intense and painful	Chronic, episodic
Lhermitte's Sign	Sudden brief, electric-shock-like sensation that runs from the back of the head down the spine; the symptom is triggered by bending the neck forward	Episodic
Trigeminal neuralgia (TN)	Caused by damage to the trigeminal nerve; stabbing, sharp pain, burning; triggered by chewing, brushing teeth, or touching the cheek	Episodic, chronic
Optic neuritis	Common MS symptom, often the initial one; pain when the eyes are moved; caused by inflamed nerve; also affects vision	Episodic, chronic
Tonic spasms	Painful spasms that cause legs or arms to move or jerk; can produce stiff or rigid muscles or limbs, which can also then become painful	Episodic, chronic

Note. Adapted from MS Society of Canada (2008)

Neurogenic Pain (see Table 9)
Also known as nerve or neuropathic pain.
- Caused by damage to a peripheral nerve or spinal cord or a dysfunction in the central nervous system.
- Can be present even in mild forms of MS.
- With MS-related demyelination, signals to the brain can become distorted by poor transmission and cause the brain to interpret certain signals as pain messages even when there is no injury.

Spasticity, caused by spinal cord damage, results in cramping, stiffness, and muscle spasms.

Comorbidities of Pain

Sleep Disorders

Sleep disturbance is a common difficulty associated with both acute and chronic pain (Field & Swarm, 2008). This can, in turn, increase other MS-related symptoms such as fatigue, depression, anxiety, and cognitive and balance difficulties.

Depression

A common symptom of MS, depression is also associated with chronic pain. One study suggests that as many as 50% of individuals with MS-related pain may have clinical depression (Diaz-Olavarrieta, Cummings, Velazquez, & Garcia de la Cadena, 1999). Additionally, inadequately treated depression can increase the perception of pain intensity (MS Society of Canada, 2008).

Anxiety

Individuals experiencing stress, anxiety, or depression report more severe pain (Maloni, 2003). In addition, it is important to address and treat pain-related fear avoidance, an anxiety-provoking thought that involves fear of movement (Field & Swarm, 2008).

Identifying stressors and treating anxiety and depression is an important component of MS pain management

Tolerance, Abuse, and Dependence

Due to the duration and frequency of visits, mental health providers are often more aware of medication misuse than the prescribing physician. Tolerance, abuse, and dependence are a concern for those being treated pharmacologically for chronic pain (Field & Swarm, 2008). These are complex issues to identify and address and justify ongoing assessment. (See Appendix 5 for a guide to assessing use of pain medication.)

Psychological Impact

The effects of pain on psychosocial functioning and emotional well-being of people living with MS is only recently becoming a focus of investigation (Kerns, Kassirer et al., 2002). However, preliminary studies suggest a similarity to the large body of existing research for non-MS specific pain. Clients with pain reported poorer mental health and greater deficits in social role and overall mental functioning compared with individuals with MS who reported no pain (Kerns, Kassirer et al., 2002).

1.6.2   Comorbidity Among Psychiatric Disorders

The co-occurrence of depression and anxiety with MS is commonplace. For example, approximately half of individuals with MS report anxiety. Fragoso et al. (2014) noted that depression, female gender, low levels of self-efficacy, disability, and stress increased the prevalence of anxiety, but only depression was an independent predictor. Independent of disability status, anxiety clearly reduces the quality of life for people with MS.

Stress and depression can trigger MS relapses

1.6.3   Comorbidity Among Cognitive Disorders

The Impact of Depression on Cognitive Performance in MS

Cognitive dysfunction frequently coexists with depression, although the exact relationship between these two factors remains unclear and appears complex. Both depression and cognitive function may stem from damage to similar neuropathological pathways, perhaps as a result of lesion location. Overall, symptoms such as psychomotor retardation, diminished interest, and/or low motivation may reduce cognitive capacity by exerting a negative effect on processing speed and working memory (i.e., the capacity to hold information in mind for further learning, mental manipulation, or processing). In MS, depression is related to attentional deficits, which can negatively affect the acquisition phase of new learning. Whether treatment of depression facilitates cognitive improvements has not been thoroughly studied in MS.

> The clinician should often slow down the rate of information presented in a session and allow time for processing

The Impact of Fatigue on Cognitive Performance in MS

Fatigue is another common symptom of MS that may impair cognitive performance (Kinsinger, Lattie, & Mohr, 2010). However, a direct relationship between fatigue and cognitive performance has not been firmly established. A related issue pertains to vigilance. That is, when concentrating very hard or working on a cognitive task for a long time, individuals with MS have been shown to have reduced vigilance and have difficulty maintaining their cognitive stamina and attention over prolonged periods. This can drain their energies, making careless errors more likely.

> Encouraging individuals to pace themselves and take short breaks can be a helpful strategy to combat cognitive fatigue

Subjective Versus Objective Cognitive Complaints

Subjective cognitive concerns are often seen in depression, and researchers have found that individuals with MS who have comorbid depression over-report cognitive difficulties (Kinsinger et al., 2010). Moreover, subjective cognitive complaints are more strongly associated with depression than objective neuropsychological functioning (Julian, Merluzzi, & Mohr, 2007). However, the degree of severity of depression may be an important variable to assess, as some research has suggested that cognitive dysfunction may appear only at higher levels of depression (Demaree, Gaudino, & DeLuca, 2003).

> Severity of depression plays a role in cognitive dysfunction in MS

Impact of Comorbid Psychiatric Disorders and Cognitive Dysfunction in Pediatric

A few studies have demonstrated higher frequency of cognitive dysfunction among children diagnosed with comorbid MS and mood or anxiety disorders compared with other children with MS. As a result, it is important for clinicians to appreciate that reduced attention and information processing speed secondary to affective disorders can adversely affect performance within other cognitive domains (Weisbrot et al., 2014). Although anxiety, mood disorders, and cognitive dysfunction may manifest secondary to neuropathological issues in pediatric MS, it is reasonable to conclude that emotional distress may be a reaction to academic and learning difficulties experienced by children and adolescents (see Table 10).

Table 10
Cognitive Dysfunction in Pediatric MST

Domains most affected in pediatric MS	Consequences of cognitive impairment in pediatric MS
Working memory Complex attention Processing speed Language and verbal comprehension Executive functioning	Failed courses Failed or poor grades Need for academic accommodations Change in college plans

1.7 Diagnostic Procedures and Documentation

1.7.1 Diagnostic Process

At first, the onset of nonspecific symptoms of MS may be misattributed to a number of other medical conditions or discounted outright. Currently, the time from the first symptom(s) to a definitive diagnosis of MS varies from a few months to a few years. It is important for mental health professionals to understand that the client who arrives at their door with an MS diagnosis may have gone through a number of medical and personal experiences that may have taxed their interpersonal and intrapersonal resources – especially self-confidence, trust in the medical field, financial resources, and social support.

1.7.2 Medical Diagnostic Procedures

Given that MS affects the brain and the spinal cord, the presenting symptoms are often varied and can be transient, and therefore these symptoms can be difficult to identify as resulting from MS. The baffling symptoms that come and go can lead to years of uncertainty and misdiagnoses. An additional source of confusion includes other conditions that have similar symptoms and may mimic MS, such as Lyme disease, rheumatic diseases, vitamin B_{12} deficiency, neuromyelitis optica, and fibromyalgia. Because of the ambiguity of these variegated disorders, initial diagnoses are often inaccurate, particularly if the patient is being evaluated by a medical professional other than a neurologist. However, consultation with a neurologist, laboratory studies, and neuroimaging can aid proper clinical diagnosis. In MS, symptoms tend to persist more than 24 hr.

The physician will take a comprehensive history to decide which tests to order. For instance, an individual may present with a specific symptom, such as vision loss in one eye or a feeling of numbness (e.g., affecting an arm or leg). If the patient also reports that several months ago or a year ago they had transient weakness in an extremity lasting more than 24 hr or are currently experiencing physical symptoms, such as difficulty with bladder control, the physician can decide if this is a central or a peripheral nervous system problem and recommend appropriate treatment.

A central feature of the diagnosis of RRMS is that lesions are disseminated both in time and in space (McDonald et al., 2007). The most recent diagnostic criteria simplify requirements for dissemination in time and space, potentially allowing for an earlier diagnosis of MS from a single baseline brain MRI if there are both silent gadolinium-enhancing and nonenhancing lesions (Milo & Miller, 2014). The diagnosis of MS by a healthcare provider includes the steps described in Table 11.

Table 11
How Is MS Diagnosed by a Healthcare Provider?

- A primary care physician rules out some of the common medical disorders that can cause symptoms (e.g., Lyme disease, vitamin B_{12} deficiency, etc.)
- Referral to a neurologist, as MS is a clinical diagnosis that requires a comprehensive evaluation that entails:
  - Review of the client's current symptom(s) and past medical history
  - Neurologic examination performed by a neurologist
  - Neurologist excludes alternative diagnoses
  - Neurologist determines which tests to order to aid differential diagnosis
- There is no test that definitively detects MS
- Medical testing may include (but is not limited to):
  - Brain and/or spinal cord imaging (e.g., MRI)
  - Examination of CSF via lumbar puncture
- The individual must experience one or more typical demyelinating events (time course and localization are considered by the medical provider); need to demonstrate dissemination of lesions in space and time

1.7.3   Common Client Responses to Diagnosis

The following responses to a diagnosis of MS are commonplace (adapted from Reitman & Kalb, 2012):

- Shock – Confusion, dissociation, going through the motions without connecting to the reality of the situation. A client may appear to accept his or her diagnosis, but may be unable to formulate questions or remember information given by professionals.
- Denial – This normal coping mechanism may initially help to mitigate psychological responses to copious amount of new information. However, some clients will ignore their diagnosis for years. They may or may not follow medical advice but will typically not attempt to optimize their health or abilities.
- Anxiety – This normal response to the unpredictability of MS may become generalized. The diagnostic process may activate previous psychological material or aggravate an existing anxiety disorder. Family members may also experience anxiety over the unpredictable impact that MS may have on their lives.
- Relief – "At least I have a name for this. Now I can figure out what to do." For those who lived with symptoms for a while before diagnosis and/or were dismissed by healthcare providers or family members, diagnosis can feel relieving and empowering.
- Grief – From diagnosis and throughout the course of the illness, a person may experience normal periods of grieving.

1.7.4   Psychiatric Diagnostic Procedures and Documentation

A clinical interview that reviews current symptoms and signs of disorders, as well as a comprehensive history, is often employed to ascertain appropriate diagnoses (see Appendix 1, "Clinical Interview – Focus on MS" for areas to be addressed in a clinical interview with individuals living with MS). Clinical assessment requires evaluation and documentation of both symptoms and psychiatric diagnostic formulations of disorders.

Symptoms (e.g., depressed mood, anxiety) are reported spontaneously by individuals or elicited through interviews, questionnaires, checklists, and severity rating scales.

Emotional disorders (e.g., major depressive, dysthymic, bipolar, anxiety, adjustment) are diagnosed according to criteria that stipulate the number and types of symptoms and their duration, intensity, and impact on functioning (see Minden et al., 2014).

Psychological evaluation is often helpful, and it is typically performed by clinicians who have experience with working with medical populations, such as clinical psychologists, neuropsychologists, rehabilitation psychologists, and health psychologists. Psychiatrists may be asked to perform a psychiatric medication evaluation and provide their psychiatric diagnostic formulation.

Mechanisms to differentiate symptoms of MS disease from depression have been proposed. Specifically, Strober and Arnett (2010) suggest that "trunk" symptoms are symptoms common to the medical condition and less reflective of depression, whereas "branch" symptoms are those that are independent of the medical condition and likely to reflect depression. Branch symptoms endorsed more often by depressed individual with MS included sense of failure, appetite changes, weight loss, pessimism, sadness, feelings of guilt, irritability, self-criticism, disappointment, and dissatisfaction. The symptoms that were common to both groups, but more severe in the depressed group, included loss of interest, dissatisfaction, crying, irritability, and self-criticism. Regrettably, there are relatively few appropriate mood measures that allow clinicians to identify and track symptoms over time.

Clinical Pearl
Cognitive Batteries

Brief, yet sensitive and specific, measures of cognitive functioning within MS still need to be developed. However, various assessment techniques and batteries have been used, and a few approaches are commonly used and appear to be the most sensitive for the detection of cognitive impairment in MS (Julian, 2011).

- The Neuropsychological Screening Battery for MS (NSBMS) was developed by the Cognitive Function Study Group of the NMSS in the United States (Rao, Leo, Bernardin, & Unverzagt, 1991). The assessment measures processing speed, attention, memory, and fluency.
- The Minimal Assessment of Cognitive Function in MS (MACFIMS) battery was developed in 2001 by an expert panel composed of psychologists and neuropsychologists convened by the Consortium of MS Centers (Benedict et al., 2002). The battery assesses processing speed, working memory, learning and memory, executive function, visual–spatial processing, and word retrieval.

2

Theories and Models

Most models of chronic illness and disability (CID) tend to focus on the individual – how the diagnosed patient is affected by the diagnosis, treatment, and progression of the disorder. This may be a reflection of the prevailing values of autonomy, independence, and individualism in many modern Western cultures. However, there are professions – such as family medicine and social work – that understand chronic illness from a systems perspective and strive to treat the whole family. When an individual is diagnosed with CID, the entire family system is affected, and the goal of treatment is to assist family members to cope effectively with changes in roles resulting from the MS diagnosis, treatment, and progression. The systemic perspective of these professions may be particularly compatible with the worldviews of clients from more traditional, collectivistic cultural backgrounds for whom family is highly valued. Mental health professionals should recognize the important role of family when treating clients living with MS.

2.1   Models of Illness and Disability

There are many ways that people living with MS, their families, and their associates may attempt to fathom the complexities of MS. Understanding how a client and significant others are conceptualizing MS will aid in the assessment and increased ability to tailor your interventions. In addition, educating clients about different models of illness and disability, and their implications, will allow your client to evaluate the effect of their beliefs on their ability to cope. Olkin (1999) described three models of disability: the moral, medical, and minority models. The biopsychosocial model is increasingly prevalent.

2.1.1   Moral Model

This model views MS as a defect caused by a moral lapse or sin. A diagnosis of MS might cause shame for the person with MS and their family and the diagnosed person and/or family members may feel responsible for causing MS. Through this lens, MS may also be viewed as a test of faith. Although, this model is not prevalent in Western culture, if it is part of a client's or family's belief system then exploration in therapy is important. Additionally, consultation with a client's religious leader will enable a psychotherapist to gain insight into how to best address coping.

2.1.2   Medical Model

This model views MS as a medical problem that results from a defect or failure of the bodily system. The person with MS is referred to as a "patient" who needs to be helped by trained professionals. In the medical model, disability is a pathology located within the individual that deviates from norm and treatment is focused on "fixing" the individual. The impact of this model can be disempowering. The expertise lies with professionals, so self-management is not encouraged and the person living with MS is not considered a knowledgeable participant in their own healthcare team.

2.1.3   Minority Model

This model defines MS-related disability as a social construct brought about by attitudes and other features of the social environment. The problems lie not with the individual but with the environment. With this model, MS-related disability becomes a socially created problem and an attribute of an individual. The solutions needed to address MS-related disabilities involve social and political fields, including universal design, education, and changes in the law.

2.1.4   Biopsychosocial Model

In 2001, the World Health Organization developed *The International Classification of Functioning, Disability and Health* (ICF) based on the biopsychosocial model. The ICF provides a coherent view of different perspectives of health: biological, individual, and social. Disability and functioning are viewed as outcomes of interactions between health conditions (diseases, disorders, and injuries) and contextual factors. Contextual factors can be external and environmental (social attitudes, architectural characteristics, legal and social structures, climate, terrain, etc.) or internal and personal (gender, age, coping styles, social background, education, profession, past and current experience, overall behavior patterns, character and other factors that influence how disability is experienced by the individual).

2.2   Minority Stress Model

The minority stress model has been used to explain health-related consequences of oppression in minority-status populations, including sexual minorities (e.g., Meyer, 1995) and African Americans (e.g., Clark, Anderson, Clark, & Williams, 1999). Briefly, the minority stress model is a biopsychosocial model that explains how various actual and perceived forms of oppression (e.g., prejudice, exclusion, aggression) from different others (out group), similar others (in group), and self can influence the onset and progression of a wide variety of disease processes (physical and emotional) via the stress response. Although it may be applicable to persons living with MS, it is important to note that the minority stress model has not specifically been investigated in this population. Nevertheless, there are important notions about the minority stress model to consider when working with anyone living with a chronic illness or disease.

For persons living with MS, stressors associated with the unpredictability of disease course include challenges to expectations from self, as well as from others. For example, physical functioning in persons living with MS may suddenly become severely compromised one day and return a few days later. How one cognitively "frames" (perceives, understands) these unpredictable changes may have a dramatic influence over how one may directly (e.g., by way of stress-related hormones) or indirectly (e.g., by way of coping behaviors) affect the disease course. Similarly, how others perceive these changes has a great influence on their own responses, which can be adaptive (e.g., offering social support) or maladaptive (e.g., expressing doubt of the symptom's authenticity) for the person living with MS.

There are two remarkable aspects of the minority stress model. First, the consequences of oppression are believed to be just as robust when oppression is perceived as when it is objectively experienced. This speaks to the strength of perceptions and schemas (cognitive frames of experience). Second, major sources of oppression include one's self and similar others. That is, internalized oppression and in-group oppression can have robust direct and indirect influence on disease processes – as much, if not more, than persecution from the majority group.

2.3   Depression

2.3.1   Depression and Psychosocial Factors

Some investigators have suggested that a relationship between physical disability and depression exists and is indirect; they note that disability affects psychosocial outcome to the degree that impairment is intrusive and personal control is threatened. Unemployment among individuals with MS is associated with a lower quality of life and is a strong predictor of a major depressive episode in persons with MS. In addition, depression is associated with reduced perceived social support. Qualitative changes in social networks and personal relationships, as a result of their disease, are often reported.

2.3.2   Depression and Neurologic Integrity

Given that MS attacks myelin and affects the integrity of nerve conduction, mood changes may be a direct neurological consequence of the disease. Mood symptoms are often found in neurological diseases when there is a subcortical component. An association between brain atrophy, as well as lesion volume (Mohr et al., 2003) and lesion location (i.e., the right temporal region or arcuate fasciculus), with depression has also been noted.

2.4   Anxiety Disorders

Anxiety is also a salient issue in MS, with perceptions of increased psychosocial stressors and decreased social support presenting as important factors in the development of an anxiety disorder, particularly generalized anxiety disorder (Korostil & Feinstein, 2007). In addition, other risk factors for the development of anxiety within MS have been identified and include female gender and a comorbid diagnosis of depression. Unexpected disrupting events in daily life serve as a reminder of MS (Kalb, 2007). For instance, among individuals with MS, those who experience relapses were shown to have the highest levels of anxiety as compared with those in remission. The assumption that anxiety emerges as a reactive phenomenon to a variety of situations is strengthened by the lack of association between anxiety and MRI abnormalities (Sá, 2008). In addition, the onset of anxiety related to needles/injections associated with treatment (i.e., self-injectable immunomodulatory drugs) may affect 50% of MS patients (Mohr, D. C., et al., 2002), although lower prevalence rates have been cited and may reflect anxious avoidance about injections rather than a frank needle phobia.

2.5   Cognitive Impairment

2.5.1   Primary Contributors to Cognitive Impairment

Primary contributions to cognitive dysfunction include brain changes

Advances in technology, such as neuroimaging, have provided insights into the association between the development of cognitive dysfunction to overall disease burden in MS (e.g., lesions, atrophy) and other specific neuropathological contributors (Julian, 2011). Cognitive difficulties can be a direct consequence of the location and extent of neuropathology and are generally not considered to be reversible.

2.5.2   Secondary Contributors to Cognitive Impairment

Secondary contributions to cognitive dysfunction include mood disorders, medications, psychosocial issues, and physical problems disrupting the individual's thinking skills

Depression, anxiety, medication effects, fatigue, and a pre-existing perfectionistic style are all factors that can contribute to one's perception of subjective concerns. The impact of these contributors can be further examined with a formal neuropsychological evaluation. Unlike primary contributors, these causes are potentially reversible and therefore present as areas that can improve with successful treatment.

3

Diagnosis and Treatment Indications

3.1 Common Points of Entry Into Psychotherapy

Clients may enter into psychotherapy at any point from early diagnosis on. However, there are three common points of entry (see Table 12).

Table 12
Issues That Inform Your Psychotherapy Treatment Planning

Newly diagnosed: 0–5 years	Normative help seeking, confusion, fear and grief, increasing premorbid psychological symptoms, re-emergence of past trauma issues.
Change in symptoms and functioning	Can represent a change in identity or loss of personal control or ability. The Stress of these changes can persist, even in those cases in which functioning improves.
Change in situation	Beginning or ending a relationship, exiting or returning to work, starting a family, and other life changes can elicit reactions that may have occurred during the initial diagnostic period. Concerns about the uncertainty of MS, finances, identity, body image as well as self-esteem issues, frustration and other emotional reactions.

Clinical Pearl
Role of Supportive Others in Medical Appointments

Individuals may be faced with stress-provoking news at medical appointments, such as being provided an initial diagnosis, updates on progression of the disorder, or feedback about test results. Having a spouse, friend, or confidant present during those medical appointments can be extremely helpful. After the physician provides feedback, clients may find that they are so emotionally overwhelmed that they do not benefit from the discussion that takes place immediately thereafter. Further, the conversation following the news typically outlines treatment options, provides useful information about supportive resources, or conveys other vital information. The presence of a trusted supportive other can help with the communication between the person living with MS and his or her healthcare provider. Their presence can also assist with reviewing the information that was provided during the appointment and help the person living with MS to formulate additional questions and a plan based on that information.

3.2   Psychological Evaluation

In addition to interviews, self-report and informant report questionnaires may be completed to identify symptoms and track effects of treatment.

3.2.1   Mood

Self-report questionnaires have been validated in MS, and we encourage you to frequently assess for depression throughout treatment. The BDI-Fast Screen (BDI-FS; Beck, Steer, & Brown, 2000) contains seven items that assess mood and negative evaluation symptoms. The measure is brief and has been shown to be valid in MS (Benedict, Fishman, McClellan, Bakshi, & Weinstock-Guttman, 2003). Moreover, the BDI-FS significantly correlates with other self-report measures and informant reports, as well. The Chicago Multiscale Depression Inventory (CMDI; Nyenhuis et al., 1995) contains three subscales (mood; evaluative/cognitive–worthlessness, failure; and vegetative) of 14 items each. The mood and evaluative scales have been shown to be reliable and valid for use in MS. Mohr, Hart, Julian, and Tasch (2007) suggested that an efficient and useful screen for depression in MS entails asking if the individual has experienced "sad mood most of the day nearly every day" for at least the last 2 weeks, and if they experienced "a loss of pleasure in most or all activities that usually gave them pleasure." They found that assessing for depressed mood and anhedonia had good sensitivity in detecting the presence of major depression, detecting 98.5% of depressed patients (Mohr et al., 2007). Relatively recently, Minden and colleagues (2014) conducted a review of psychiatric assessment measures in an effort to provide evidenced-based guidelines and noted support of the two-question tool to screen for depressive disorders, as well as the Beck Depression Inventory.

3.2.2   Suicide Risk

Although disability itself does not appear to be a factor that places individuals at risk for harming themselves, individuals with comorbid depression and MS have a considerably increased risk of suicide. In addition to direct questioning about suicidal ideation, intention, means, plans, attempts, and self-harm gestures, the clinician is encouraged to assess for suicide risk factors in MS. Risk factors include depression, social isolation, lower income, and younger age, as well as male sex, disability, a sense of hopelessness, and loss of control.

3.3   Emotional Components of Living With MS

Living with MS may involve certain predictable emotional components

In addition to the reaction to the initial diagnosis, there may be normative and predictable emotional components to living with MS (see Table 13).

Table 13
Common Emotional Reactions to Living With MS

Grief	From diagnosis and throughout the course of the illness, a client may experience periods of normal grieving.
Resentment	Response to the unpredictability and the financial and logistical impact for people with MS and their family members alike.
Guilt, shame, and self-blame	For a person with MS this may arise owing to difficulties controlling bodily functions, fulfilling family and occupational roles and obligations, or a belief that they may have caused the disease or an increase in symptoms. For associates and family members, it may stem from the ability to do things that the person with MS cannot do or ambivalence with offering support and/or providing caregiving.
Fear and distrust	The stressors of the unpredictability of MS, the possibility of progression and increased disability, the potential for medication failure and side effects, the potential loss of income, and the high expense of healthcare can lead to fear of loss and distrust of the body, healthcare providers, and significant others.
Anger and frustration	Response to lack of options, accessibility, support, and other stressors of living with MS. This can be misdirected toward significant others and professionals who are trying to help.
Confusion and overwhelm	Response to the multifaceted aspects of the disease, the treatments, and navigating life with MS.

Note. Adapted from Reitman and Kalb (2012).

3.4 Cognitive and Psychiatric Disorders Impeding Psychotherapy and Medical Treatment

3.4.1 Cognitive Difficulties

Cognitive deficits become problematic for clients living with MS when these symptoms begin to interfere with daily functioning and treatment (e.g., difficulty making progress in therapy), as well as when clients or loved ones become distressed by these deficits. One of the more common tasks for mental health professionals is to help determine when cognitive deficits experienced by a client living with MS may be organically associated with disease progression (i.e., brain lesions); when they may be related to MS treatment (e.g., medication); when they may be secondary to a mood disorder; when they may be part of normative aging; or when they may be a consequence of a combination of factors. One of the major roles of the mental health professional is to know when to refer to a professional who can conduct a more thorough and specialized evaluation, such as a neurologist, neuropsychologist, psychiatrist, occupational therapist, or speech pathologist. Although a neuropsychological evaluation can be a helpful method for teasing apart contributing factors of cognitive dysfunction, a few things for a mental health professional to keep in mind include:

- Cognitive deficits such as forgetfulness and word-finding difficulty may be related to MS fatigue.
- Cognitive difficulty associated with depression is usually accompanied by hopelessness and helplessness about oneself, the world, and the future.
- Mood disorders in general are often associated with identifiable, precipitating events (e.g., loss of physical functioning, financial difficulties, interpersonal difficulties) – all of which, unfortunately, are prevalent among persons living with MS.
- Mental health professionals should always be aware of cognitive changes that may be associated with recent changes in a client's medication or treatment regimen.

3.4.2   Cognitive Dysfunction and Neurobehavioral Problems

Cognitive dysfunction can hamper gains in treatment. Specifically, clients may encounter difficulty attending to important treatment-related information during an appointment with their medical provider. Likewise, clients may experience problems sustaining or shifting their attention during psychotherapy. Memory problems, such as difficulty retrieving information, can challenge the carry-over of information over time. Reduced executive functions, such as poor initiation and problems with prioritizing, problem solving, and reasoning, can affect treatment-related decision making. Neurobehavioral problems can also occur; individuals can experience difficulties regulating behavior and affective responses, which may be associated with frontal-limbic system dysfunction. These neurobehavioral symptoms (i.e., diminished insight, impulsivity, apathy, disinhibition, emotional dysregulation) can cause problems with motivation, engagement in therapy tasks, compliance with treatment recommendations, safety, compensatory strategy use, employment, and interpersonal relationships.

3.4.3   Depression and Pain

The ability of an individual with MS to self-manage his or her condition and its effects on daily living will be influenced by depression and pain. Depression can affect self-management through its impact on energy, motivation, concentration, self-efficacy, and interpersonal functioning. Indeed, depression has been implicated in reduced adherence to disease-modifying therapies and other interventions. Individuals with MS and comorbid chronic pain tend to be inactive and report diminished self-efficacy for symptom management.

3.4.4 Sleep Disturbance and Psychiatric Comorbidity

Sleep disturbance can contribute to mood or anxiety symptoms, frequently observed increases in irritability and aggression, behavioral dysregulation, and reduced engagement in treatment. Sleep fragmentation and fatigue can also significantly affect cognitive functioning. Individuals may show reduced alertness, inattention, and other cognitive problems secondary to sleep disturbance. In turn, cognitive dysfunction can negatively influence the quality of engagement in treatment.

3.5 Medication Issues

Many factors must be considered and ruled out before initiating medications in order to correctly attribute symptoms and avoid unnecessary or unhelpful treatments when working with neurologic populations (Taber, Hurley, & Yudofsky, 2010). For instance, multiple symptoms shared by both major depressive disorder and MS can impede proper diagnosis (Paparrigopoulos, Ferentinos, Kouzoupis, Koutsis, & Papadimitriou, 2010), and this is why depression continues to be underdiagnosed and undertreated in individuals with MS. Similarly, depression may occur with treatment by some disease-modifying regimens, such as interferon beta-1b (although this continues to be debated). Therefore, continuous monitoring of medication-related mood/behavior symptoms, prevention, and treatment is critical when working with individuals with MS.

Psychiatric effects of disease-modifying interventions, symptomatic therapies, and corticosteroids used in MS deserve further investigation. An accurate and complete diagnostic impression and treatment plan requires recognition of the underlying neuropathology and an understanding of the confluence of genetic, environmental, and psychosocial influences.

Potential sources of physical, cognitive, and neuropsychiatric symptoms are:

- MS
- Comorbid medical and neurologic conditions
- Medication effects, including polypharmacy
- Social factors (e.g., abuse, neglect, interpersonal conflict)

Special considerations may need to be taken when prescribing medications to individuals with neurologic diagnoses because they are often more sensitive to medication side effects (Taber et al., 2010):

- Limit polypharmacy by prescribing as few medications as possible.
- Implement a slower medication titration.
- Frequently and persistently reassess dosage levels.
- Remain vigilant for signs of toxicity and drug interactions, especially additive anti-cholinergic or sedative effects.
- Minimize the use of agents that impair cognition, increase sedation, increase disinhibition, or impede neuronal functioning (e.g., benzodiazepines, anticholinergics, seizure-inducing agents, antidopaminergics).

3.6   Psychological Difficulties of Learned Helplessness and Secondary Gain

3.6.1   Learned Helplessness

Introduced by Martin Seligman in 1973, the concept of learned helplessness suggests that certain populations, such as the chronically ill, who are routinely exposed to uncontrollable aversive illness events risk the development of learned helplessness. Peterson and Seligman (1987) proposed that learned helplessness could be related to detrimental health outcomes. One study indicated that learned helplessness is associated with negative health indicators in the MS population; specifically, it predicted more active disease and greater functional and social disability (McGuiness, 1996). McGuiness further suggested that because of the unpredictability of MS, the focus of treatment should be enabling self-management and control of those areas of the disease that can be controlled.

3.6.2   Secondary Gain

A client may consciously or unconsciously utilize the MS diagnosis as a way of avoiding responsibilities or unpleasant activities. This can become very contentious in relationships. Posing the question, "What would your life be like if you began to feel better?" can aid with assessment.

3.7   Prioritizing Problems and Needs

The SARI model (Frederick & McNeal, 1999; Phillips & Frederick, 1995) was originally developed as a guide for working with clients exhibiting post-traumatic and dissociative symptoms. This model has not been applied to the CID or MS populations, and its use here is not suggestive or indicative that there is any similarity between these psychiatric symptoms and CID or MS. However, as it offers a useful guide for structuring therapy, especially for those clients whose MS diagnosis and treatment have activated previous trauma material, we have adapted the model for this publication. For clients with no prior trauma or mental health difficulties and in a short-term therapy frame, the entire focus will be on the first two areas.

S – Safety and Stabilization: Establishing internal and external safety; needs and safety assessment, crisis intervention, accessing resources, education and referrals. The focus is on assessing the client's situation, ability, support systems, coping skills and healthcare resources and assisting clients in comprehending the effect of MS on their lives. If capable, strengthening the client's movement toward self-mastery.

A – Activation of Psychological Stressors: Focus on stressors that may be impacting health and developing inner resources needed to resolve them. This includes interventions for stress and pain reduction. MS may not be the focus of therapy at this point.

R – Resolution: If there is a trauma history, MS symptoms, disease progression, and/or healthcare may evoke traumatic material that can result in dissociation, fragmentation, high levels of activation, or decompensation. Traumatic experiences need to be reprocessed so that stressors either do not evoke psychological and somatic reactions or the client is able to independently and rapidly settle these reactions.

I – Integration and Internalization: If inner conflict, fragmentation, and instability have been issues in health impairment, the focus should be integration and increased stabilization. The goal is progress toward the ability to either self-manage or consistently participate in health and wellness decisions that will increase quality of life.

3.8   Focus of Psychotherapy

Psychotherapy can focus on health and wellness issues, or it can address clinical concerns such as depression, anxiety, or suicidal ideation. A focus on health and wellness will primarily address the MS diagnosis, developing and working with a treatment team, symptom management, and the client's wellness plan (see Table 14). A focus on clinical concerns will include assessment, coping skills, adaptation, as well as individual, group, and family psychotherapy.

3.8.1   Health and Wellness

Considerations for patient health and wellness involve various aspects:
- Treatment decisions – Clients may ask the therapist to help them decide whether or not to take medications or which medications to use. The decision lies with the client. *The role of the therapist is to assist the client with problem solving, reducing anxiety, increasing resources, and solidifying trust in the treating physician.*
- Treatment team development – Ideally, a client will have a good working relationship with a neurologist and primary care provider. *The role of the therapist is to assist the client in evaluating the effectiveness of his or her healthcare team, evaluating the level of trust that the client has in the treating physicians, and facilitating referrals to healthcare professionals.*

Mental health professionals can play an integral role in building a comprehensive healthcare team

- Symptom management – Management of fatigue, pain, stress and the psychological impact of fluctuating MS symptoms. *The role of the therapist is education, intervention, and referral.*
- Cognitive functioning – This may require consultation with a neuropsychologist. Recording sessions, making notes, writing down assignments, providing a clear written treatment plan, and sending reminders may improve the success of the therapy sessions. *The role of the therapist is to assess clients' ability to self-manage both their medical and psychological symptoms and treatment.*

Table 14
Concepts of Wellness

Wellness is the goal – not cure	Pursuing health and wellness activities may or may not result in changes in symptoms. Clients may get disheartened and unmotivated if they do not see noticeable improvement.
Quality of life	Utilizing coping skills, accommodations, interventions, and creativity to maintain or increase the perceived quality of life.
Balance and pacing	Pacing is structuring activities to incorporate time and fatigue management. Balance is utilizing abilities, self-care, and resources to maximize quality of life.
Learning to adapt	Employing innovative ways to accomplish goals. This can include use of mobility aids, accommodation at work, and universal design at home.

Developing a Wellness Plan

A mental health professional can assist clients in developing a wellness plan

There are identifiable phases incorporated in developing a self-care/wellness plan. However, different authors often use different terms when discussing wellness. Dr. Werfel has utilized the following model and the associated terms since 1997 (see Appendix 2 for a detailed description). This is not a linear

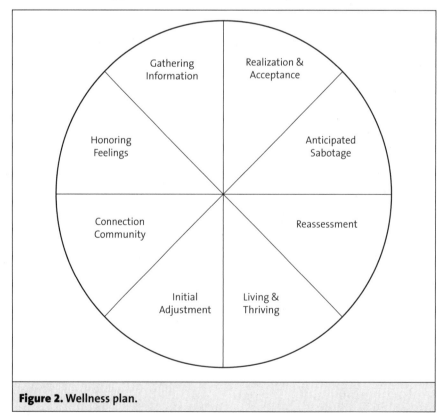

Figure 2. Wellness plan.

process, as indicated by the chart in Figure 2, and phases may need to be revisited and updated numerous times to reflect changes in the disease process, in healthcare advances, and in the person's resources.

3.8.2   Clinical Focus

The clinical focus when treating patients with MS should take into account the following points:

- **Abuse** – People with disabilities can experience physical and emotional abuse from caregivers, and they are vulnerable to financial manipulation and theft. *The role of the therapist is evaluation, intervention, and mandatory reporting.*
- **Body image** – MS does not feel sexy. Even those with hidden symptoms may feel unattractive.
- **Caregiver stress** – The role and responsibilities of a partner will change dramatically if disability increases. A partner may not be willing or physically or emotionally able to assume a caregiver role. Additionally, even a willing and able caregiver can encounter compassion fatigue. Figley (1995) defined compassion fatigue as the combination of compassion stress and burnout. Compassion stress is defined as a natural consequence resulting from helping or wanting to help a person who is suffering. It can result in anger, frustration, guilt, loneliness, illness, and exhaustion. Burnout, characterized by mental and physical exhaustion, cynicism, ineffectiveness, and depersonalization, is the result of long-term involvement in situations that are emotionally demanding. *The role of the therapist is increasing awareness and communication and providing support, self-care tools, and referrals.*

  > **Both professional and familial caregivers are susceptible to compassion fatigue**

- **Communication skills** – Unpredictable or hidden symptoms are difficult to explain to others. However, the capacity to clearly communicate about abilities and struggles to healthcare providers, caregivers, family and friends, through written or spoken language, is essential (see http://livingwell.mscenter.org).

  > **Speaking about MS and the associated stressors is challenging for many people**

- **Disclosure** – Disclosure is a decision that clients with MS will encounter at work and with each new person and situation. The Americans with Disabilities Act laws do not prevent discrimination. *The role of the therapist is problem solving, skill building, anxiety management, and referral.*
- **Encourage independence** – Focus on self-mastery and self-efficacy whenever possible.
- **Family** – MS is considered a family disease because it affects the entire family. Co-joint or family sessions are often necessary and almost always helpful.
- **Financial decisions** – *The role of the therapist is assisting in evaluating financial health and providing resources and referrals.*
- **Focus on strength** – Many people who are living with MS are able to contribute at a high level to their families and/or work environment. *The role of the therapist is maximizing the client's strengths and abilities and utilizing these strengths to build mastery.*

  > **MS will significantly affect the finances of a client and family**

- **Identity formation and self-esteem** – Diagnosis and living with MS affects identity, body image, and self-esteem. Feeling different, less capable, dependent, unattractive, and boring is common. Fluctuating and hidden symptoms increase identity formation difficulties.
- **Increase body awareness and connection** – Many people who are not living with CID are relatively unaware of their body. MS symptoms, especially pain, often result in even further dissociation from the body. Body awareness will optimize self-care, mobility and stress, pain and fatigue management.
- **Interaction with the medical community** – Frustration and disappointment with medical options and providers will often be a focus of therapy. *The role of the therapist is to facilitate communication with healthcare providers. This may include advocating for a client or educating a healthcare provider.*
- **Occupational decisions** – How or whether to enter, remain in, or exit the workforce are difficult and complex decisions. Evaluations from neuropsychologists or occupational therapists can facilitate these decisions.

Parents' reluctance to discuss the effects of MS on the family can result in children experiencing insecurity and instability

- **Parenting** – Reitman and Kalb (2012) state that recent studies have reported no significant, long-term psychological or behavioral difficulties in children who have a parent with MS. However, they note that parents need to model coping by providing children with information about MS and enable their children to ask questions and explore their feelings. In addition, roles can shift as children may either need to become more independent or assume more responsibility in the household or with the care of a parent who has increasing disabilities. Further, parents may be less available or more irritable because of discomfort, fatigue, or psychiatric symptoms.
- **Psychoeducation and coaching** – High-functioning clients, with no prior mental health issues, might not need traditional psychotherapy, but rather education, encouragement, and support.
- **Psychiatric diagnoses** – (see Section 1.7.4)
- **Quality of life** – Evaluation of current quality of life is important to include in any initial evaluation. *The role of the therapist is to provide interventions and encourage utilization of activities that will maintain or increase perceived quality of life.*

A diagnosis of MS often affects relationships

- **Relationships** – People with MS sometimes become less involved in activities that they previously enjoyed either because of physical or emotional challenges or because of time, energy, or financial constraints. Emotional distance may develop if the person with MS either assumes that others do not want to hear about or cannot understand his or her experience, or assumes that others are either disinterested or overwhelmed.
- **Sexuality** – MS can affect sexual desire and performance; likewise, poorer body image can affect one's sense of desirability. *The role of the therapist is to foster open discussion aimed at reducing shame and increasing communication with the client's partner, as well as to provide resources and referrals.*
- **Strengthen coping skills** – Cultivate humor, creativity, tenacity, and build on prior self-mastery.

3.9   Psychosocial Adaptation

Clinical Pearl
Evaluating Coping

Helping clients evaluate and utilize their natural coping mechanisms, increasing their coping flexibility and social support, engendering resilience, and tailoring interventions to their coping style will facilitate psychosocial adaptation.

Smedema, Bakken-Gillen, and Dalton (2009) describe psychosocial adaptation as the process through which individuals move toward an optimal state of adjustment to CID. If adjustment is achieved, the client is able to value his or her existing abilities and acknowledge his or her limitations, effectively solve problems, and negotiate in the external environment. Psychosocial adaptation appears to not only affect the quality of life for people with MS but may also impact MS symptoms. For example, Schwartz, Coulthard-Morris, and Zeng (1996) found that "people who feel that they can choose or create environments suitable to their psychic or physical conditions report less global MS-related fatigue and less fatigue-related distress" (http://www.ncbi.nlm.nih.gov/pubmed/8607741). Conversely, Mohr (2007) reports that "poor coping and low social support have been implicated as aggravating the relationship between stress and MS exacerbation" (http://www.ncbi.nlm.nih.gov/pubmed/17503132).

> Helping clients evaluate and utilize their natural coping mechanisms will facilitate psychosocial adaptation.

The importance of cultivating social support is highlighted in the literature as an important component of psychosocial adaptation. McDaniel, Hepworth, and Doherty (1999) stated that the quality of a person's social relationships appears to be the most powerful psychosocial factor in health and illness. In a review of the literature of people with MS, Livneh and Martz (2012) found that perceived social support corresponded with decreased depression and was linked with better perceived quality of life and life satisfaction.

Psychosocial Stressors With MS

MS can present multiple stressors relative to identity, relationships, and social interactions. Two potential stressors are *microaggression* and *microinvalidation*. Coined by Chester M. Pierce in 1970 and researched extensively by Derald Wing Sue, the term *microaggression* originally described verbal aggressions toward racial/ethnic groups. Sue (2010) has since expanded this definition to everyday verbal, nonverbal, and environmental slights, snubs, or insults, whether intentional or unintentional, which communicate hostile, derogatory, or negative messages to target persons based solely on their marginalized group membership. Sue states that the most detrimental forms of microaggression are usually delivered by well-intentioned individuals who are unaware that they have engaged in harmful conduct toward a socially devalued group.

> People living with CID can become marginalized in an able-bodied dominant society and suffer the effects of microaggression

Research indicates that microaggressions have a powerful impact on psychological well-being and affect the standard of living of marginalized groups by creating inequities in healthcare, education, and employment (Sue, 2010).

This is illustrated by the assumption that people with physical challenges will not be hard-working, capable employees. In addition, people with MS who may have encountered microaggression owing to their ethnicity or sexual orientation may now have an additional stressor of microaggression focused on disability. Further, people of color or homosexuals may be more hesitant to attend an MS support group for the first time, for example, because of previous experiences of microaggression in other settings.

Sue (2010) defines microinvalidations as verbal comments or behaviors that exclude, negate, or nullify the psychological thoughts, feelings, or experiential reality of a person. A common example for people living with hidden MS symptoms is the response, "Oh, but you look so good, it can't be that bad" when they seek support.

Developmental Stressors

There may be a significant difference between how adolescents might manage an MS diagnosis versus someone in their 50s

There are different developmental tasks at each stage of life (see Table 15). In addition, coping strategies and skills can change with life experience. Life experience may bring increased mastery and self-awareness, but it can also result in less flexibility and tenacity.

Table 15
Developmental Stressors

Stage and task	Average person	Include for Individuals with MS	Coping
Adolescence			
Identity, peer acceptance and relationships, sexuality, bodily changes, attaining independence, future plans, self-esteem[a]	Preoccupation with body and appearance Testing limits and abilities Rebelling against authority Experimentation[a]	Disruption to social and emotional development, delay in independence Identity formation separate from diagnosis/disability[a]	Youth may be able to compensate for less mastery with optimism, flexibility, and tenacity
Young adulthood			
Intimacy Vocational goals Independence Social responsibility Socialization[a]	Do I want a higher education/ career? Do I want to have a long-term partner/ have children? Where do I want to go out tonight? What do I want to wear? Friends, work, fun, self-efficacy is the focus	Will I be able to pursue an education/career? Will I be able to find a life partner /raise children? Will I have enough energy to go out? Will I be able to walk in these heels? When/if should I tell my boss/dates/ new friends? Increased health focus	May retain flexibility, open-mindedness, optimism, and increase development of self-awareness, self-confidence, and mastery

Table 15 (continued)

Stage and task	Average person	Include for Individuals with MS	Coping
Middle adulthood			
Further occupational development Relationship commitment and family	Where do I want to live? What house/ apartment do I want to live in? Do I want	Where will I be able to live – temperature, accessibility, healthcare? Will I be able to	May have increased awareness of abilities and mastery based on life
Economic stability Care of parents Stable living situation Helping children gain independence[a]	to change occupation/job? When do I want to retire? Where do I want to go on vacation? How do I want to support my children?	keep my job/work until retirement age? Will I be able to change jobs? Where am I able to go and enjoy? Can I help my children?	experience; may have less flexibility, optimism, willingness
Later adulthood			
Retirement planning Increased focus on physical and cognitive ability and healthcare Supporting aging life-partner[a]	How and where do I want to spend my retirement/later years? Health, wellness, and maintaining abilities become the focus	Where can I live? Increased concern about personal financial and energy resources and healthcare and not burdening family[a] Age-related health issues may complicate MS treatment and symptoms	May have an established support network, increased awareness of inner and external resources, less confidence in physical abilities Those with MS may have developed enough mastery with MS symptom management that they are better able to cope with age-related physical challenges

Note. [a]Adapted from Falvo (2009).

Stressors Associated With a New Diagnosis and Disease Progression

We previously described the stressors associated with a new diagnosis; these include getting and understanding the diagnosis, treatment decisions and access, and potential change in self-esteem, ability, finances, and activities. The stressors of living with MS also include the unpredictability of symptoms and progression, involvement with the healthcare system, symptom management and relationship, occupational and financial challenges. Additionally, if the disease progresses, managing new symptoms and interventions, adjusting to decreased ability and independence, and the need for mobility aids will further strain both psychological and financial resources and coping mechanisms.

Models of Psychosocial Adaptation

Linear or stage models of psychosocial adaptation are frequently proposed in the adaptation literature. These models describe the stages that one has to progress through to achieve adaptation, with each stage predicated on the successful completion of the prior stage (Smedema et al., 2009). Although helpful in conceptualizing adjustment, linear models may not be entirely relevant to those living with MS.

The process of adaptation to MS can look quite different from client to client and adjustment may be part of an ongoing process. For example, if initial symptoms are quite mild, a person might begin medication and continue on with their life without giving MS too much thought until years later when either more intrusive symptoms or another life change requires a different form of adaptation. Conversely, another person, also with mild symptoms, may adapt by researching the disorder, pursuing wellness, and seeking support immediately after diagnosis; however, this person will still need to continue to adapt if symptoms progress. Olkin (1999) says of living with a disability: "We have the task of constantly adjusting and then when we think we have adjusted, adjusting again." (pp. 241-242).

3.10   Coping

> **Clinical Pearl**
> **Coping With MS**
>
> Coping with MS is a complex endeavor. One client stated in the initial session, "It seems like just when I got past my fear and sadness, accepted that this may not get better, and started using a scooter, I became able to walk better again and discovered that it was a relapse, not a progression. It's like living on a roller-coaster."

A general definition of psychological coping is based on individuals gaining control over symptoms, understanding how their world has changed, understanding their own reactions to events, mourning, and psychologically reconstituting (Allen, 2003). However, definitions – based on the premise that one can understand, adjust, and move on – do not address the unpredictability of MS and the reality that some symptoms resist management. Wortman and Brehm (1975) theorized that repeated failure at tasks would lead to learned helplessness. Therefore, if the goal is gaining control of MS, failure can lead to a sense of helplessness. An alternative goal is to assist the client in being able to control what is controllable; developing and/or maintaining psychologically, physically, and spiritually healthy behavior. Framing the goal of therapy as making it easier to live with MS is more likely to result in self-efficacy rather than helplessness.

Coping Strategies

Since Lazarus began investigating coping strategies in the 1960s, research has not shown evidence that any one coping strategy is superior in all situations (Carver, Scheier, & Weintraub, 1989; Suls & Fletcher 1985). Rather, effective coping appears to be influenced by a number of factors, including perceived control, cultural resources, and coping flexibility. However, research has indicated that plan-based active, problem-solving coping modes result in lower overall psychosocial distress, lower levels of depression, and higher life satisfaction (Livneh & Martz, 2012). Schwartz and Rogers (1994) posit that effective coping is characterized by flexibility rather than by the use of specific styles or strategies. They define coping flexibility as "the ability to recognize when what one is doing is not working and to shift in a purposive trial and error manner to new approaches" (p. 58). This requires a repertoire of coping strategies, which can be developed and tested with the support of a psychotherapist.

Allen's (2003) categorization of coping strategies as *avoidant, psychological,* and *instrumental* provides an easily understandable frame to discuss coping with clients. Pakenham's (2012) work on coping strategies with the MS population notes similar categories of *problem-focused* and *emotion-focused* strategies, which can include both avoidant and psychological elements. He additionally notes *meaning-focused* and *benefit-finding coping.* Pakenham (2012) reported that poorer adjustment related to reliance on avoidance and emotion-focused coping. Additionally, Pakenham and Cox (2009) found that benefit-finding coping was related to better adjustment. (See Appendix 3 for full chart and explanations.)

Resilience

Clinical Pearl
Encouraging Resilience in Clients

Positing the question, "what can we learn from this?" after a failure may counter helplessness by helping the client to set more attainable goals.

Case: A young woman feared that she would not be able to have a social life because of MS-related fatigue. To illustrate her belief, she described having to call in sick to work after going out with coworkers the previous evening. The client and therapist were able to evaluate this scenario and generate alternatives. In this particular case, she had not slept well the night before so she was already tired before going out. A light drinker, she drank more than she typically would, went to sleep much later than usual, and had another poor night's sleep. While discussing these extenuating factors, she became aware that she could make different choices. Going forward, she was able to join in enough social activities with coworkers to make solid friendships at work. She also initiated activities that were better suited to her abilities.

The therapist can engender resilience by encouraging clients to gradually build mastery, through interventions and assignments

Resilience, a component of coping, involves utilizing personal assets and resources to enable self-protection, overcoming the adverse effects of risk exposure, and adjusting to the effects of a physical disability or impairment (Craig, 2012; Rutter, 1985). Therefore, supporting and increasing a client's resilience is an important component of psychosocial adaptation (Bonanno & Mancinni, 2008).

Self-efficacy specific to managing MS-related challenges seems to be related to better adjustment than generalized self-efficacy (Dennison, Moss-Morris, & Chalder, 2009). Chwastiak and Ehde (2007) found that a *protective factor* from familial, social, and professional support reduces negative risks. Additionally, the *challenge model* purports that successful or resilient outcomes are dependent on levels of risk exposure (Craig, 2012). Craig explains that successfully managing a lower-level symptom will increase motivation to attempt to manage more difficult symptoms. Conversely, if past interventions have failed, the resulting feelings of hopelessness may lead to lower motivation to try new interventions.

Perceived Control and Coping

According to the coping matching hypothesis (or goodness of fit hypothesis), events that are perceived as controllable are best met with active, problem-focused coping strategies, while events perceived as uncontrollable are best met with emotion-focused coping strategies (Forsythe & Compas, 1987; Zankowski, Hall, Klein, & Baum, 2001). The key term is *perceived*. While certain events or conditions may appear clearly under one's immediate control or not, the perception of controllability of most situations is in the eye of the beholder. One of the major tasks for mental health professionals working with individuals living with MS is to determine how the unpredictability of symptom progression is perceived – that is, what aspects of MS are experienced as within or outside of the client's personal control and how the client emotionally, cognitively, and behaviorally responds to that uncertainty.

Bandura's social cognitive theory (1997) is a good model to help determine how two factors – *self-efficacy expectancies* (the extent to which one believes one can perform a certain action) and *outcome expectancies* (the extent to which one believes the environment will respond favorably to one's efforts) – may be associated with emotional, cognitive, and behavioral responses to certain events, situations, and conditions (see Figure 3). Although the direction of influence among expectancies, mood, behavioral responses, and perceptions is

	High self-efficacy expectancy	Low self-efficacy expectancy
High outcome expectancy	Hope High motivation	Disappointment Low motivation
Low outcome expectancy	Frustration Low motivation	Dejection Low motivation

Figure 3.
How self-efficacy and outcome expectancies relate to mood and motivation. Based on Bandura's social cognitive theory (1997).

still under investigation, Bandura hypothesizes a complex system of reciprocal determination among these and related factors. The good news for mental health professionals about reciprocal determination is that interventions may be effectively targeted at any number of points along the chain of cognitions, moods, behaviors, beliefs, and values.

Culture and Coping

According to Lazarus and Folkman's stress and coping model (1984), intra- and interpersonal resources influence our perceived ability to cope with an event through our appraisal of the event as stressful, challenging, or neutral. The degree of an event's perceived controllability, therefore, may be largely influenced by the information, values, attitudes, and beliefs that are afforded to us under the umbrella of "culture."

For a number of sociohistorical reasons, individuals of social minority status (i.e., low socioeconomic status, ethnic minorities) may perceive many of life's events as generally outside of their personal control. One common finding in the stress and coping literature is that persons of minority status tend to utilize religious coping more than other individuals do (Pargament, 1997). Research has delineated five styles of religious coping that tend to run along the lines of problem-focused and emotion-focused coping (see Table 16).

In general, use of the collaborative style of religious coping has shown the best results. However, spiritual surrender may be helpful when there remain few objectively controllable aspects to one's experience. For individuals who have a Christian belief system, spiritual surrender has been positively associated with reduction in anxiety and anger (Pargament, Smith, Koenig, & Perez, 1998).

For most modern, secular mental health professionals religion is an uncomfortable topic to address (sexuality and finances are similarly "taboo" subjects). Moreover, clients from a minority religious tradition may not feel

Table 16
Religious Coping Types

Religious coping type	Description	Problem-focused or emotion-focused
Self-directing	God expects me to take control, be responsible, etc.	Problem-focused
Collaborative	God is a partner in the coping process	Problem-focused
Deferring	Only God can influence the situation.	Emotion-focused
Pleading	Depending on God to solve the problem	Emotion-focused
Spiritual surrender	Giving over to God, but retaining responsibility	Emotion-focused and problem-focused

Note. Adapted from Pargament (1997).

comfortable talking about such personal issues to an "outsider." However, failure to assess the role of religion in a client's coping repertoire may result in a loss of vital information. Moreover, it may set an unhealthy precedence of silence and non-disclosure about taboo topics. The mental health professional's approach to assessing religious coping should be frank and direct, using the perspective of the client's religious tradition to explore issues of uncontrollability, uncertainty, and other existential issues. We recommend consultation with an appropriate religious authority when a mental health professional is not familiar with a client's religion.

MS can be a major disruption to the balance of social roles in the family. From a family therapy perspective, when one member is diagnosed with MS, the entire family is affected. The concept of family is of central value to many cultures, and family members often serve as the only acceptable source of social support. This is understandable, especially among families that have sociocultural histories of oppression from outsiders as a product of war, immigration, indentured servitude, etc. However, family as sole source of social support may be very limiting, particularly when one requires specialized information and assistance, as in the case of MS. Another problem with family as the sole source of social support is that certain types of support from family can be both helpful and deleterious. In particular, *solicitous* support in response to pain or disability – usually from spouses and close family members – has been shown to be invalidizing for clients, largely because it is believed to reinforce a client's helplessness, inactivity, and pain behavior (e.g., Itkowitz, Kerns & Otis, 2003; Kerns, Rosenberg & Otis, 2002).

Experiential factors associated with time can also affect coping with MS. These factors include age, developmental level, and time since diagnosis. These are cohort effects. One good example of a cohort effect is the finding that younger women diagnosed with breast cancer psychologically respond less favorably than older women do (e.g., Kroenke et al., 2004). The data suggest that a breast cancer diagnosis for a younger woman may be developmentally disruptive to more areas of life than the same diagnosis in an older woman – for example, younger women often are dealing with relatively newer marriages, raising young children, or starting a profession. More mature women, on the other hand, may be more accepting of health problems as a normative part of aging, or they may have developed more effective coping skills as a function of time and maturity.

Similarly, time since diagnosis is an important factor associated with coping with chronic illness. For many individuals living with chronic illness, time since diagnosis may yield mastery and acceptance. In the cancer literature, for example, survivorship has been shown to facilitate meaning making, and some women actually report psychological growth after having experienced cancer diagnosis and treatment. Unlike cancer and most other well-studied chronic illnesses, however, it is important to remember that MS does not have a predictable, linear course. Therefore, the effects of time since diagnosis may not be as important as experience with certain symptoms or frequency of setbacks.

Coping Styles

Understanding the monitor–blunting coping style (Miller, 1991) can assist both therapist and client in determining how to most effectively contend with the vast amounts of available, yet inconclusive, information about MS and treatments. *Monitors* attempt to lower stress by information gathering but can get overwhelmed by the amount of material. *Blunters* cope by minimizing the information they receive and may avoid getting the information that they need to make decisions about treatment. In one study with a non-MS population, Williams-Piehota, Pizarro, Schneider, Mowad, and Salovey (2005) found that matching healthcare messages to coping style could increase adherence to medical protocols.

3.11   Social Support

An MS client's social support network is a vital resource that should be periodically assessed by the treating mental health professional. There are several types of social support: *informational support* provides the facts and figures we made need to make informed choices; *instrumental support* includes the financial and practical help we need to live; *affiliative support* provides feelings of belongingness; and *emotional support* provides the empathy and positive regard we require for a better quality of life. In addition, there are a variety of sources of social support: family, friends, physicians, employers, community, church, etc. (see Schwarzer, Dunkel-Schetter, & Kemeny, 1994; Schwarzer, Knoll, & Reickmann, 2003).

Difficulties with social support come in many forms. One common difficulty is the inability to effectively ask for assistance. It is not uncommon for a client to lack the life experience and social skills required to effectively ask for assistance, and he or she may require assertiveness training in order to obtain what is needed. In addition, MS often strikes individuals during the time in their lives when they are in the roles of parent and/or breadwinner. From a developmental perspective, it may be especially difficult for someone who has these role expectations to ask for assistance.

A second common difficulty with social support is that individuals often have the false belief that one social support source (usually a partner or a parent) can provide all the support one needs *all the time*. Certainly, this faulty expectation can readily be challenged and changed through psychoeducation. In the United States, for example, while we expect physicians to provide accurate informational support, they are usually not allowed enough time with patients to provide meaningful emotional support. Likewise, while we may expect emotional and instrumental support from spouses, this source of support may not be the best place to obtain medical information.

A third, closely related, challenge with social support is helping clients identify which sources of support are most beneficial. It is maladaptive, for example, to expect a good friend who does not own a car to provide transportation to one's weekly occupational therapy meetings. That good friend may be better suited to provide emotional support, while someone else may be better outfitted to provide transportation (a form of instrumental support).

Clinical Pearl
The Importance of Evaluating Support Systems and Screening in High-Risk Community Settings

Mental health professionals can assist clients living with MS to identify their needs and then identify who in their social network is best equipped to provide that support.

3.12   Referral Issues

Difficulties that can complicate referral include:
- *Shortage of qualified professionals*: Local professionals may not have experience with MS.
- *Insurance coverage*: Clients may not have insurance or adequate coverage, or their insurance may not cover the treatment or hold contracts with experienced professionals.
- *Financial constraints*: Clients may not be able to afford the co-payments or other out-of-pocket expenses.
- *Accessibility*: Offices may not be accessible or transportation is an issue.
- *Lack of follow-through*: Client may be resistant to the referral or experience symptoms that may interfere with treatment, such as fatigue, depression, and or cognitive difficulties.
- *Insurance requires physician-generated referral*: Communication with treating physician about purpose of referral will decrease complications.

4

Treatment

4.1 Methods of Treatment

4.1.1 Integrative Healthcare

The Consortium of Academic Health Centers for Integrative Medicine defines integrative medicine as an approach that focuses on the whole person, is informed by evidence, and makes use of all appropriate therapeutic approaches, healthcare professionals, and disciplines to achieve optimal health and healing. Working in an integrative way enables both mental and physical health professionals to provide high-quality care. In addition to conventional medical and mental health interventions, integrative medicine can include complementary and alternative medicine (CAM) and mind–body interventions. In the literature, the terms *CAM* and *mind–body interventions* are sometimes either used interchangeably or mind–body interventions are included as a subset of CAM. However, for the purposes of this publication we use separate rubrics based on the training of mental health professionals.

The size and composition of an MS treatment team can vary widely depending on medical need and access to specialists. It is not unusual for a person with MS to be primarily treated by either a neurologist or a primary care physician who consults with a neurologist. However, depending on the needs of the client, the treatment team also could include psychologists, psychotherapists, occupational and physical therapists, social workers, primary care physicians, ophthalmologists, gynecologists, urologists, pain management specialists, clinical nurse specialists, psychiatrists, and CAM practitioners.

4.1.2 Medical Treatment for MS

Disease-Modifying Therapy (DMT)
Regardless of whether individuals are newly diagnosed or received their diagnoses some time ago, they face important treatment decisions that can have long-term implications. Clearly, the use and selection of DMT is an important consideration in treatment-related decision making (NMSS, http://www.nationalmssociety.org/Treating-MS/Medications). Current preventive DMTs primarily target attacks and aim to reduce both the frequency and severity of these attacks (Wingerchuk & Carter, 2014). These treatments have variable safety and tolerability profiles. Injectables are safe; by contrast, many newer agents do not have the same safety profile. DMTs have been shown to reduce

the risk of physical disability, and can diminish the number of active brain lesions visible after MRI. However, at present there is no identifiable way to predict better outcome with a specific drug for an individual. A comprehensive understanding of the benefit–risk profiles of DMTs is necessary to establish logical and safe treatment plans (Cree, 2014):

- The route and frequency of administration
- Tolerability and likelihood of treatment adherence
- Adverse effects
- Risk of major toxicity
- Special considerations: pregnancy-related risks

Collaborative decision making between a person with MS and his or her medical provider is encouraged. There are numerous and salient issues to be addressed in treatment selection (Wingerchuk & Carter, 2014):

- Recent MS activity (recent attack frequency, severity, and recovery)
- The degree of neurological impairment
- The "lesion burden" (and the presence of active enhancing lesions) evident on brain and spinal cord MRI
- Concomitant medical conditions and medications
- Individual preferences for injection type and frequency
- Avoidance of certain adverse effects
- Drug availability and cost

There are 13 U.S. Food and Drug Administration (FDA)-approved DMTs for RRMS with varying degrees of efficacy for reducing relapse risk and preserving neurological function, but their long-term benefits are not firmly established (Wingerchuk & Carter, 2014; see Table 17). Among these, four interferon beta preparations and glatiramer acetate are immunomodulatory drugs approved for relapsing MS. The interferon beta and glatiramer acetate treatments have favorable long-term outcome safety profiles and monitoring requirements are known to be minimal. These treatments have been shown to have comparable efficacy (Wingerchuk & Carter, 2014), as research has indicated that they reduce the clinical relapse rate by about one-third and moderate the development of new brain MRI lesions over periods of 1–3 years for both clinically isolated syndromes (Comi et al., 2009) and relapsing MS (Panitch et al., 2002). They are as typical first-line treatment choices, despite the advent of oral therapies. Peginterferon beta-1a was approved by the FDA in August, 2014. Three oral DMTs are approved for relapsing MS, namely, fingolimod, teriflunomide, and dimethyl fumarate/BG-12.

Clinical Pearl
Discussing Treatment Options

Individuals living with MS benefit from a discussion about treatment decisions that bolster:

- Identifying what they hope to achieve with treatment
- Providing education about realistic expectations

- Understanding the benefits and risks of the treatment(s)
- Reviewing the primary concerns that they would like addressed (e.g., bladder problems, capacity to continue working, emotional control, independence in walking, etc.)
- Exploring their worries about what MS will do to their body and life
- Uncovering their general perspectives, including apprehensions, about treatment
- Discussing the perspectives of important others regarding treatment (e.g., how they may view the decision to take or not to engage in the treatment)
- Exploring cultural viewpoints about their healthcare provider, medications, alternative therapies, asking for assistance, and the impact of gender and/or social roles on treatment-related decisions

Table 17
Disease-Modifying Therapies for MS

Disease-modifying therapy	Brand name	Year approved	Route	Frequency
Interferon beta-1b	Betaseron	1993	Subcutaneous	Every other day
	Extavia	2009	Subcutaneous	Every other day
Interferon beta-1a	Avonex	1996	Intramuscular	Weekly
	Rebif	2002	Subcutaneous	Three times per week
Peginterferon beta-1a	Plegridy	2014	Subcutaneous	Every 14 days
Glatiramer acetate	Copaxone	1997	Subcutaneous	Daily or 3 times per week
Natalizumab	Tysabri	2004, 2006	Intravenously	Every 4 weeks
Fingolimod	Gilenya	2010	Oral	Daily
Teriflunomide	Aubagio	2012	Oral	Daily
Dimethyl fumarate	Tecfidera	2013	Oral	Twice a day
Alemtuzumab	Lemtrada	2014	Intravenous Infusion	5 consecutive days initially and then 3 consecutive days 1 year later
Glatiramer acetate	Glatopa (generic form of Copaxone)	2015	Subcutaneous	Daily
Mitoxantrone	Novantrone	2015	Intravenous Infusion	Every 3 months

Researchers continue to explore the efficacy of current treatments as well as to investigate novel therapies. Despite the advances that have occurred, some researchers have noted the need to establish therapies that robustly slow or halt progressive forms of the disease or potentially repair or regenerate areas of the CNS impacted by MS (Wingerchuk & Carter, 2014). There are conflicting data regarding the association between depression and treatment with some disease-modifying drugs, particularly interferon beta-1b (see Table 18).

Clinical Pearl
Treatment Considerations

When deciding to engage in treatment (e.g., DMTs, symptom management medications, supplements), clients are encouraged to work collaboratively with their healthcare professionals to:
- Understand the types of side effects that may be experienced.
- Clarify the estimated time that side effect(s) will persist; clarify whether it is a short-term side effect that will be experienced while adjusting to the medication or a long-term side effect that remains during the entire time the individual is taking the drug.
- Identify ways that the healthcare provider plans to minimize the risk of developing a side-effect.
- Establish a plan on how they will be monitored for side effects, as well as how often monitoring appointments will occur.

Table 18
Risks and Potential Adverse Effects of DMTs

Interferon beta preparations	Injection-site reactions Flu-like symptoms Elevated enzymes in liver function tests Leukopenia Depression
Glatiramer acetate	Injection-site reactions Benign systemic reaction (dyspnea, palpitations)
Mitoxantrone	Cardiac toxicity Leukemia
Natalizumab	Infusion reactions Progressive multifocal leukoencephalopathy
Fingolimod	Bradyarrhythmia Macular edema Herpes virus infections (varicella zoster virus)
Teriflunomide	Teratogenic risk Hepatotoxicity
Dimethyl fumarate/BG-12	Flushing (dose-related) Gastrointestinal symptoms and gastrointestinal side effects Leukopenia
Alemtuzumab	Secondary autoimmunity

Table 19
Symptom Management and Psychosocial Implications

Symptom	Description	Psychosocial implications	Treatment
Fatigue: primary (neurologic)	Overwhelming lassitude or tiredness that can strike at any time of day, regardless of activity level or amount of sleep, and is often exacerbated by heat.	Inability to carry out activities at home and at work (a major factor in early departure from the workforce and changes in family roles). Fatigue of this magnitude affects mood and quality of life. Invisible symptom that is easily misinterpreted by others as laziness or disinterest.	Rehabilitation: Address secondary contributing factors (primary sleep disturbance, nocturia [neurogenic bladder], pain, spasticity, periodic limb movements); refer to PT (energy conservation; moderate aerobic exercise; mobility aids) and OT (work simplification/energy conservation; nap schedule; use of assistive devices at home/work; cooling strategies/devices). Medications: Amantadine, modafinil, armodafinil, fluoxetine.
Fatigue: secondary (resulting from disturbed sleep; depression; extra exertion due to impairments; medications)		Inability to carry out activities at home and at work (a major factor in early departure from the workforce and changes in family roles). Fatigue of this magnitude affects mood and quality of life. Invisible symptom that is easily misinterpreted by others as laziness or disinterest.	Rehabilitation: Address secondary contributing factors (primary sleep disturbance, nocturia, pain, spasticity, periodic limb movements); refer to PT (energy conservation; moderate aerobic exercise; mobility aids) and OT (work simplification/energy conservation; nap schedule; use of assistive devices at home/work; cooling strategies/devices).

Table 19 (continued)

Symptom	Description	Psychosocial implications	Treatment
Heat and temperature sensitivity	Many people with MS experience a temporary worsening of their symptoms when the weather is very hot or humid or they run a fever. Activities including sunbathing, getting overheated from exercise, or taking very hot showers or baths can have the same effect. For example, some people notice that their vision becomes blurred when they get overheated – a phenomenon known as *Uhthoff's phenomenon*. These temporary changes can result from even a very slight elevation in core body temperature (one quarter to one half of a degree). An elevated temperature further impairs the ability of a demyelinated nerve to conduct electrical impulses. Some people with MS notice that symptoms, particularly spasticity, become worse in cold weather.	Restrictions imposed by temperature sensitivity on capacity to engage in exercise and to participate in leisure activities; impact on tolerating climates in work environments.	Stay in an air-conditioned environment during periods of extreme heat and humidity. If an air conditioner is needed to help minimize the symptoms of MS, the cost of this equipment may be tax deductible if the physician has written a prescription for it. Use cooling products such as vests, neck wraps, and bandanas, during exercise or outdoor activity, or pre- and post-cool. Wear lightweight, loose, "breathe-able" clothing. Icy drinks or popsicles can provide temporary relief. Use an oscillating fan during indoor exercise. Exercise in a cool pool (<85°F/30°C).

Table 19 (continued)

Symptom	Description	Psychosocial implications	Treatment
Bladder and bowel symptoms	Failure to store (urgency, frequency, incontinence, nocturia/neurogenic bladder). Failure to empty (urgency, hesitancy, double voiding, feelings of incomplete emptying). Combined failure to store/failure to empty (urgency, hesitancy, double voiding, feelings of incomplete emptying). Constipation.	Fear of drinking liquids; anxiety over loss of control; fear of leaving vicinity of bathroom. Embarrassment/shame; fear of incontinence during intercourse; increased fatigue due to interrupted sleep. Fear/embarrassment related to catheter use.	Interventions: Check for UTI; scheduled voiding; avoidance of diuretics. Intermittent self-catheterization (ISC); may require indwelling catheter. Bowel training; adequate fluid intake; high-fiber diet; exercise; medications (bowel): polyethylene glycol, psyllium, docusate, bisacodyl.
Spasticity (can range from relatively mild to quite severe)	Phasic spasms (flexor or extensor). Sustained increase in muscle tone.	Spasticity can increase fatigue and interfere with functioning at home and at work. Spasticity can interfere with sexual activity and comfort. Oral medications may increase fatigue and weakness. Surgical implantation of pump in abdomen can be frightening. Severing of tendons is irreversible.	Rehabilitation: Rehabilitative PT: stretching, gait assessment, and balance training, if needed. Medications: Oral medications: baclofen, tizanidine, dantrolene, clonazepam, gabapentin, levetiracetam (phasic spasticity), clonidine, diazepam. Intrathecal baclofen pump: OnabotulinumtoxinA injections into individual muscles (FDA-approved for upper limb spasticity). Surgery.

Table 19 (continued)

Symptom	Description	Psychosocial implications	Treatment
Ambulation/mobility problems	Ataxia. Weakness. Impaired balance.	Resistance to use of mobility aids. Perceptions of self: damaged; weak; "giving in" to MS. Others' perceptions: less intelligent; less competent.	Rehabilitation: Referral to PT: mobility aids; exercise. Medications: Dalfampridine (FDA-approved for this use) to improve walking speed.
Tremors	Gross tremor is characterized by wide back-and-forth motions, usually of the arms or legs. Intention or action tremors are activated when a person reaches for something. When tremor is severe, it can prevent a person from eating, writing, speaking clearly, or walking.	Loss of control – severe tremor is a major threat to independence. Increased fatigue caused by medications.	Rehabilitation: Referral to PT for balance/coordination exercises; referral to OT for tools; weights on limbs, eating or writing utensils. Medications: Propranolol, clonazepam, hydroxyzine, primidone, isoniazid, topiramate, buspirone, ondansetron, gabapentin.
Dysarthria and dysphonia	Poorly articulated, slurred, hypophonic (low volume) speech.	Slurring can be misinterpreted as drunkenness or lack of intelligence. Slow, slurred, and/or dysphonic speech interferes with communication and interactions, and increases the risk of isolation.	Referral to S/LP for assessment as soon as changes are noted or reported; exercise program; training with augmentative or alternative communication devices, if needed.

Table 19 (continued)

Symptom	Description	Psychosocial implications	Treatment
Visual symptoms are common in MS. Optic neuritis is the presenting symptom in 25% of MS patients.	Optic neuritis: temporary loss or disturbance of vision, often accompanied by pain; may also cause a "blind spot" (scotoma) in center of vision; nystagmus.	Visual symptoms can threaten independent functioning (e.g., driving), increase fatigue, and interfere with activities at work and at home.	Training in visual compensation, environmental modifications, adaptive equipment, as needed.
Sexual dysfunction is common in people with MS and is important to assess because patients may be reluctant to self-report. Secondary contributing factors: Fatigue; spasticity; bladder/bowel problems; sensory changes; mood issues interfere with sexual activity. Tertiary (resulting from disability-related attitudes/feelings)	Impaired arousal; sensory changes; reduced vaginal lubrication; erectile dysfunction; inability to achieve orgasm. Tertiary factors: feeling unattractive; unable to attract a partner; believing that sexuality is incompatible with disability.	Significant impact on gratification, self-esteem, self-confidence; difficult/ embarrassing to discuss with health-care providers. Significant impact on all intimate relationships: Sexual activity can be difficult, exhausting, painful, and unsatisfying. Lack of arousal can be misunderstood and resented by partner. Learning new ways to be intimate can be frightening and difficult. Partner may become disinterested in, or uncomfortable with, their disabled partner. Person with MS may be reluctant to become intimate with new partner.	Interventions: Education; evaluation; counseling; sexual aids to enhance stimulation. Effective management of other (secondary) issues. Psychological: individual and couple's counseling and education. Medications: Men – oral medications: sildenafil, vardenafil, tadalafil; injectable or insertable medication: alprostadil. Prosthetic devices. Women: lubricating substances; enhanced stimulation.

Table 19 (continued)

Symptom	Description	Psychosocial implications	Treatment
Sensory symptoms (paresthesias) Primary pain Central neuropathic pain Trigeminal neuralgia Dysesthesias Retro-orbital pain Secondary pain (musculoskeletal)	Paresthesias—numbness, tingling, pins and needles. Trigeminal neuralgia – a stabbing pain in the face that can occur at any time during MS, even as an initial symptom. While it can be confused with dental pain, this pain is neurologic in origin.	Heightened distress; people with MS may interpret their pain as a serious deterioration of their condition.	No treatment required unless interfering with function; medication if necessary; referral to PT/OT if necessary. Medications: For central neuropathic pain and trigeminal neuralgia – carbamazepine, oxcarbamazepine, gabapentin. For dysesthesias – tricyclics, pregabalin, gabapentin; lidoderm patch. Other – topical application of capsaic acid cream. Psychological: Behavioral self-management (mindfulness, meditation); hypnosis, cognitive behavior therapy; CAM; and massage, relaxation, humor, music, and distraction. Medications for retro-orbital pain – high-dose IV steroids. Musculoskeletal pain: Referral to PT: gait and balance training; assessment of all seating (home, automobile, work, and wheelchair/scooter). A multidisciplinary pain clinic.

Note. PT = physical therapy. OT = occupational therapy. UTI = urinary tract infection. S/LP = speech and language pathologist. IV = intravenous. Adapted from Kalb (2012).

Treatment of Acute Relapses

Evidence-based recommendations regarding the treatment of acute relapses of MS have been documented in great detail elsewhere (Ontaneda & Rae-Grant, 2009). In summary, studies have demonstrated that corticosteroids increase the speed of recovery from MS relapses but long-term improvement of disability has not been demonstrated. There is limited support regarding the efficacy of intravenous immunoglobulin (a sterile solution of concentrated antibodies extracted from healthy donors that is administered into a vein) and plasma exchange in acute MS relapses; therefore, they are considered second-line treatments when there is poor response to corticosteroids or when corticosteroids are contraindicated.

Symptom Management (Medications, Rehabilitation, Other Interventions)

Due to the multiple sites in which it is possible for MS lesions to develop, there is wide variability in symptom presentation. The symptoms described in Table 19 may frequently manifest in MS and potentially exert influence on quality of life and psychosocial functioning.

Quality of life, including psychosocial functioning, can be significantly influenced by MS

> **Clinical Pearl**
> **Self-Perception**
>
> MS is a very physical disease, but it can also tax one's self-concept. While the individual did not choose MS, he or she can choose how to think and address the challenges in their life. The symptoms associated with MS can be used as justification for disengaging from activities a client needs or wants to do. Therefore, the individual should be encouraged to manage the impact of the symptoms by doing whatever he or she is capable of doing. Therapists can help clients avoid comparing what they can now do with what they could once do.

4.1.3   Complementary and Alternative Medicine

In the United States, approximately 75% of people with MS use some form of CAM (http://www.nationalmssociety.org). The terms *CAM* and *mind–body interventions* are often either used interchangeably or mind–body interventions are included with CAM. However, we define CAM as complementary and alternative interventions that are typically outside the area of practice of mental health professionals. The National Center for Complementary and Integrative Health (NCCIH) has also defined CAM: *Complementary* refers to using a non-mainstream approach together with conventional medicine. *Alternative* refers to using a non-mainstream approach in place of conventional medicine ((NCCIH, n.d.).

CAM interventions can range from well-researched, safe, and effective to experimental, ineffective, and potentially harmful methods. The most common MS-related symptoms treated by CAM are pain, insomnia, mobility challenges, fatigue, and stress (see Table 20).

People with MS pursue CAM interventions because conventional treatment was not effective, because they have heard anecdotal reports of the utility

Table 20
Most Frequently Utilized CAM Interventions for MS

Acupuncture	A component of traditional Chinese medicine. Practitioners stimulate specific points on the body, usually by inserting thin needles through the skin, at specific points. Preliminary studies indicate that acupuncture may improve MS-related anxiety, depression, dizziness, pain, numbness, spasticity, bladder difficulties, and weakness.[a,b,c]
Chiropractic	There is anecdotal evidence that people with MS have experienced some symptom relief with chiropractic manipulation.[b]
Cooling therapy	Specific to the treatment of people with MS. Sensitivity to heat can result in weakness, fatigue, spasticity, tremor, coordination, visual, cognitive, urinary, sexual, and walking difficulties and speech disorders. Limited research studies have shown an improvement of these symptoms with cooling therapy. Methods for treatment can be a cold shower, or a cooling vest, bandana, or suit. However, the cooling vest and suit appear to bring the most relief.[b,c]
Diets	Most of the dietary studies in MS involve polyunsaturated fats. Dr. Swank's 50-year longitudinal study, treating people with MS with a low saturated fat, high polyunsaturated fatty acid diet plus supplements, indicated that those on his diet had less frequent and severe attacks, reduced overall impairment, and decreased death rate. Although this study does not meet current standard criteria, it appears safe and the recommended diet may be beneficial.[b]
Hydrotherapy	A low-risk water exercise that can include adapted swimming, deep and shallow water aerobic exercise, and balance and flexibility training. It can be helpful in improving flexibility, strength, balance, coordination, and endurance and in decreasing pain, depression, and fatigue for those living with MS. In one study with people with MS, the effects were superior to those of the equivalent non-aquatic exercise program (Castro-Sánchez et al., 2011).
Vitamins, minerals, and supplements	Surveys of people with MS indicate that the use of supplements is one of the most common forms of CAM. Increasing evidence points to a connection between low vitamin D levels and MS. Some supplements are now recommended for preventing or treating a limited number of conditions.[a]
Marijuana	Promising results have been obtained in preliminary studies of the use of marijuana or its derivatives to treat MS-related spasticity and pain. Health Canada, the drug regulatory agency for Canada, has approved the use of the cannabis-derived drug Sativex for MS-related symptoms.[c]
Massage therapy	Includes many different techniques in which practitioners manually manipulate the soft tissues of the muscles. Studies with other medical conditions show possible benefits for depression, anxiety, spasticity, constipation, and pain.[b,c]

Table 20 (continued)

Prayer	The healing power of prayer has been studied for many years. Variable results have been obtained in studies of the effects of prayer on other medical conditions. Anxiety and stress, which may occur with MS, appear to be reduced by prayer.[a]
T'ai chi and qi gong	Practices from traditional Chinese medicine that combine specific movements or postures, coordinated breathing, and mental focus. May provide both a less strenuous exercise and some of the benefits of meditation. Studies suggest that it might help people with MS decrease muscle stiffness, improve walking, and help with emotional and social functioning.[b]
Yoga	Increasing numbers of MS experts note that yoga, with its emphasis on relaxation, breathing, stretching, and deliberate movements, is a good choice of exercise. [a,c] One 6-month controlled study found that yoga intervention showed significant improvement in measures of fatigue in people with MS. (Oken, Kishiyama, Zajdel, et al., 2004). Other studies have provided suggestive results with pain, depression, anxiety, memory, concentration, spasticity, and overall sense of well-being.[a]

Note. [a]Rocky Mountain MS Center, n.d., (http://www.mscenter.org/resources/publications). [b]Bowling & Bowling, n.d., (http://www.neurologycare.net). [c]NMSS (http://www.nationalmssociety.org/Treating-MS/Complementary-Alternative-Medicines).

of CAM, or because of a doctor's referral (Olsen, 2009). Although much of the scientific research on CAM and MS is preliminary, there are enough anecdotal reports of benefits from CAM that the NMSS and some MS clinics offer CAM programs and interventions. Allen Bowling, a noted neurologist, has authored two books on MS and CAM and maintains a website with updated information (http://www.neurologycare.net), and the Rocky Mountain MS Center has gathered a substantial amount of information that it publishes on the website http://www.mscenter.org.

4.1.4   Neuropsychiatric Treatment (Psychopharmacology)

Neuropsychiatry is the subspecialty of psychiatry that addresses disorders at the interface of neurology and psychiatry. Neuropsychiatric symptoms are often present in MS, even in the early stages of the disease (Paparrigopoulos et al., 2010). Neuropsychiatric symptom constellations often present in neurologic populations include:
- Depression (includes apathy)
- Psychosis (includes disturbances of perception and/or thought)
- Agitation (includes anxiety and mania)
- Emotion dysregulation and behavior problems (includes aggression and impulsivity)
- Cognitive disturbances (includes dementia)

Table 21
MS-Specific Treatment Information for Neuropsychiatric Symptoms

Neuropsychiatric symptom	Treatment
Depression and apathy	Paparrigopoulos and coworkers (2010) note that there is only one randomized controlled trial of an antidepressant, namely, desipramine, in MS patients (Schiffer & Wineman, 1990). Open-label trials and case reports have given promising results for selective serotonin reuptake inhibitors (SSRIs) and monoamine oxidase inhibitors, and electroconvulsive therapy (ECT) may be helpful in the management of severe treatment-resistant depression despite a 20% risk of exacerbation in MS symptoms following ECT. The interferon beta medications carry warning labels stating that they should be used with caution by anyone who is depressed or has a history of depression. Sidhom and colleagues (2014) noted that although initial studies have reported cases of suicide and depression in individuals treated with interferon beta, none of the randomized controlled trials using standardized and validated measures of depression showed a significantly increased risk of depression in those treated with interferon beta (Wilken & Sullivan, 2007). Although research has failed to show a strong link between depression and the interferon beta drugs used to treat MS, these medications decrease levels of the chemical serotonin in the brain – and decreased serotonin can affect mood. Worsening of mood disorders in MS was not shown in other studies for those individuals treated with interferon beta for a long period (Porcel et al. 2006). That is, the presence of major depression is not an absolute contraindication to treatment with interferon beta, although neurologists are vigilant of the potential onset of depression in all individuals with MS, whether they are on disease-modifying treatment or not.
Bipolar disorder	According to Paparrigopoulos et al. (2010), in the absence of published treatment studies, anecdotal reports suggest management with mood stabilizers (lithium, valproate, carbamazepine), antipsychotics, and benzodiazepines, whereas in the case of steroid-induced mania, lithium prophylaxis and reduction of steroid dose may allow clinicians to avoid steroid treatment discontinuation. Sidhom and colleagues (2014) emphasized that the risk of exacerbation of psychiatric disorders using corticosteroids, which are not constant and occur more frequently in case of a discontinuous treatment, should not delay their use. They noted that manifesting psychiatric symptoms could still be treated with mood stabilizers, neuroleptics, or antidepressants with simultaneous steroid taper. A somewhat related issue is pseudobulbar affect syndrome, also referred to as pathological laughing and crying. Minden and colleagues (2014) note that a combination of dextromethorphan and quinidine may be considered.

Table 21 (continued)

	Antidepressants and L-dopa have been traditionally used to treat pseudobulbar affect (Arciniegas, 2005). SSRIs are recommended as first-line pharmacotherapy, although if SSRIs are ineffective or poorly tolerated, tricyclic and novel dual-action antidepressants, venlafaxine, duloxetine, mirtazapine, lamotrigine, levodopa, and dextromethorphan/quinidine have been reported as second-line treatments (Paparrigopoulos et al., 2010).
Anxiety	Anxiolytic drugs used in the general population may be used to treat anxiety in individuals with MS (Korostil & Feinstein, 2007).
Psychosis	A relationship between lesions in temporal brain regions and psychosis has been noted in the literature. The psychosis-inducing effects of medications such as steroids and interferons have been noted, although there are no published treatment trials. On the basis of anecdotal evidence, small-dose atypical antipsychotics are generally preferred, mainly because of the reduced risk of extrapyramidal side effects (Paparrigopoulos et al., 2010).
Cognition	Limited research has been produced regarding potential cognitive improvement with disease-modifying treatments (interferon beta-1b, interferon beta-1a, and glatiramer acetate). Specifically, in a meta-analysis (Galetta, Markowitz, & Lee, 2002) comparing all disease-modifying drugs, only three out of 21 studies entered in the analysis could provide useful cognitive data. Among these, interferon beta-1a, based on a single, well-designed and executed treatment trial was favored. Trials of acetylcholinesterase inhibitors used in Alzheimer's disease, such as donepezil, have been tried in individuals with MS who also have cognitive dysfunction. The majority of these studies have consisted of small, open-label investigations. In a randomized, double-blind, placebo-controlled trial of 69 cognitively impaired MS patients, Krupp and colleagues (2004) found marginal benefits from donepezil on a single cognitive domain – although further examination of the role of this medication and others in cognitive dysfunction remains necessary.

Table 21 includes information gleaned from the literature on treatment of neuropsychiatric symptoms within MS. The extant research on psychopharmacologic treatment in MS is limited. Additional information on treatment within the general category of neurologic disorders has been detailed elsewhere in greater detail (e.g., see Taber et al., 2010).

4.1.5   Interdisciplinary Rehabilitation in MS

Rehabilitation aims include minimizing impairment, increasing productivity, providing environmental support, reducing social and other barriers, and enhancing personal coping strategies

Rehabilitation is a problem-solving educational process aimed at reducing disability and enhancing participation. Multiple reviews document that gains in the health, physical fitness, and quality of life of people with MS are related to engaging in rehabilitation therapies. An interdisciplinary rehabilitation team comprises rehabilitation professionals (e.g., physiatrists, neurologists, ophthalmologists, physical therapists, occupational therapists, speech therapists, vocational rehabilitation specialists, rehabilitation psychologists, neuropsychologists, and social workers). According to the American Psychological Association (Division 22), rehabilitation psychology is the study of the application of psychosocial principles in working with persons with physical, cognitive, developmental, or emotional disabilities (American Psychological Association, Division 22, n.d.). Rehabilitation is designed to be individually focused, time-limited, and functionally oriented, with the overall goal of maximizing activity and participation (social integration). Rehabilitation interventions are often introduced early in treatment to enhance functional capacity, support the individual's capacity to perform activities, and reduce risk for losing important abilities or independence. Impairments in MS are problems with body structure and function (strength, coordination, balance, spasticity, memory, urinary urgency), which result in activity limitation (such as difficulties executing everyday tasks, mobility, self-care, incontinence, pain, cognitive deficits, and restriction in societal participation – impact on work, driving, family, finances). Rehabilitation therapies address prevention of decreased functioning, facilitate remediation (restoration), and bolster compensation (alternatives, modifications, or accommodations).

In MS, many symptoms are responsive to rehabilitation efforts, although it is a constantly changing process given the variability of symptoms that can occur throughout the disease process. From a psychological perspective, participating in rehabilitation provides individuals with a way to take charge of their disease and learn strategies to cope, and perhaps remediate, problems. In addition, family and supportive others are often encouraged to be involved and can benefit from that inclusion.

4.1.6   Cognitive Rehabilitation

There are two primary approaches to cognitive rehabilitation: (1) *remediation*, which entails re-training of specific skills and (2) *compensation*, which focuses on learning new methods to address weaknesses and "work around" a cognitive difficulty. There is accumulating evidence that suggests that significant improvement is possible with both approaches. Cognitive reserve refers to both passive reserve, which reflects past indicators of brain reserve, such as IQ, educational and occupational attainment, and childhood enrichment activities, as well as active reserve, which refers to current enriching and cognitive-stimulating activities that keep the brain active and healthy (e.g., leisure activities, exercise, etc.). To this end, speech therapists, occupational therapists, and neuropsychologists can assist individuals implement cognitive compensatory strategies and identify environmental modifications to improve performance in daily functioning. Research has shown that individuals with MS who possess high passive and/or active reserve appear to be healthier and experience higher levels of well-being. The neuropsychologist, as well as rehabilitation therapists (e.g., speech therapists, occupational therapists), can review strategies to compensate for weaknesses and discuss ways to promote active cognitive reserve. Cognitive reserve has broad implications for understanding cognitive resilience. Given that cognitive reserve refers to the idea that intellectual enrichment is associated with cerebral efficiency and therefore neuropsychological performance, it may buffer individuals against the long-term cognitive effects of the disease and possibly even protect against the transition from relapsing-remitting to progressive disease course.

4.1.7 Psychological Interventions

When a person living with a diagnosis of MS initiates psychological treatment, mental health professionals must realize that – no matter how long ago the diagnosis was received – the person before them has actively responded to the news through a filter made up of pre-existing thoughts, beliefs, values, and past personal experience. One way to look at this experiential filter is to understand that it is likely influenced by the client's identity, which consists of various cultural units such as age, gender, education, race, ethnicity, sexual orientation, language, and religion. Another way to conceptualize a client's responses to MS is to think of them as coping.

Clinical Pearl
Initial Assessment of Effect of MS on Client's Life

For most mental health professionals, a generally good start to effective treatment is a thorough assessment – using the lens of the client's cultural identity – of how MS has changed the client's life and how the client has responded to those changes.

Psychotherapy

In general, any form of psychotherapy that involves compassionately listening and helping a client sort out the complex emotions, daily life challenges, and decisions that come with an MS diagnosis can be helpful. However, psychotherapy and psychological interventions can offer much more than support. Research suggests that face-to-face behavioral interventions may decrease inflammatory disease activity, such as relapse rate. Therefore, behavioral interventions have the potential to modify the disease process itself (Heesen et al., 2012).

People with MS may be resilient and high functioning but still need help from a psychotherapist

Most of the research on psychotherapeutic interventions with MS has focused on cognitive-behavioral therapies. There also is some evidence highlighting the value of education, goal setting, homework assignments, and multidisciplinary team support (Malcomson, Dunwoody, & Lowe-Strong, 2007). However, there is not a single recommended therapeutic approach or theoretical model for MS. Therefore, this section will contain a review of models that are more commonly described in the literature for CID. A therapist can draw on interventions from a number of different models to best meet the needs of an individual client.

Psychoeducation

Reitman and Kalb (2012) defined psychoeducation as "a supportive educational process designed to enhance people's understanding of the disease, adaptive coping strategies, and available resources" (p. 39) and listed it as a key component of ongoing psychosocial support for someone living with MS.

It can also be used in conjunction with other models of psychotherapy. Psychoeducation may be especially useful for the newly diagnosed, but due to the changing nature of both the disease and people's lives, education is an ongoing process.

The psychoeducational process can both enhance therapeutic bonding and be utilized as an assessment tool. Asking clients what they know about MS, how MS affects their body, and what they know about MS treatments, will enable the therapist to gauge the level of knowledge, the reaction to the information, and whether the client is utilizing reliable resources. For example, information gained in an Internet chatroom can be inaccurate and disconcerting and may have led to misconceptions and distress. In addition, psychoeducation can reduce stress by normalizing a client's experience and offering concrete information and tools.

Effective use of psychoeducation requires an understanding of a client's coping style (e.g., is he or she a *monitor* or *blunter*?). The therapist can give an assignment to review therapist-provided resources that can be discussed in the next session. However, not all clients have the ability or desire to independently review the material. Conversely, some clients keep themselves apprised of the latest research developments in the MS literature and will bring these to therapy, to discuss.

Cognitive-Behavioral Therapy (CBT)

CBT combines cognitive and behavioral therapeutic approaches to modify maladaptive thought processes that are believed to contribute to the onset and/or maintenance of emotional and behavioral problems. Originally designed to treat people in emotional distress, CBT has been used to effectively treat individuals living with the direct and indirect consequences of chronic illness, like MS (e.g., Askey-Jones, David, Silber, Shaw, & Chalder, 2013; Dennison & Moss-Morris, 2010; Mohr, Boudewyn, Goodkin, Bostrum, & Epstein, 2001; Thomas, Thomas, Hiller, Galvin, & Baker, 2006).

There are several cognitive behavioral therapies, including exposure therapies, stress inoculation training, cognitive processing therapy, relaxation training, dialectical behavior therapy (DBT), and acceptance and commitment therapy (ACT). While some clinicians are cognitively oriented (e.g., cognitive restructuring), others are more behaviorally oriented (e.g., *in vivo* exposure therapy). Interventions such as imaginal exposure therapy combine both approaches. According to Persons and Davidson (2010), most therapists who consider CBT as their preferred modality of therapy use a combination of CBT methods in practice, most of which contain the following six phases of treatment:
- Pretreatment assessment
- Reconceptualization

- Skills acquisition
- Skills consolidation and application training
- Generalization and maintenance
- Posttreatment assessment follow-up

Given its relatively brief, systematic, behavioral approach and solution-focused nature, CBT is readily amenable to traditional forms of research evaluation. A number of studies have demonstrated CBT to be at least as effective as antidepressants in treating mild and moderate depression and anxiety. Studies also show that a combination of antidepressants and CBT can be effective in treating major depression. Moreover, CBT for the treatment of MS has been readily adaptable to both individual and group settings, and the techniques have been successfully adapted for self-help applications. In addition, CBT for persons living with MS has been successfully adapted for alternative treatment modalities, such as therapy provided via telephone or by computer (e.g., Mohr et al., 2000). This is especially fortunate, given that persons living with MS, for many reasons, experience difficulty traveling to standard therapy appointments.

There are numerous CBT manuals and workbooks readily available on-line and in bookstores.

CBT and Depression

Lewinsohn's model (1974) of major depressive disorder describes mood disorder as resulting from a lack of participation in pleasurable activities, often the consequence of poor social skills. From this perspective, a classic CBT approach for a person living with MS who is experiencing depression would be to first assess how much pleasurable activity the client is experiencing. This would be assessed through direct interviewing, and a client would also be given homework in the form of a journal or chart to note any and all pleasurable activities experienced during the week between sessions. The chart would elicit, for example, a description of each activity, the context under which it was experienced (e.g., location, time of day, duration), and a Likert-type assessment (usually using a scale from 0 to 5) of the client's mood immediately before and after each activity. After gathering the information, the client and therapist will review the homework together, identify the type and number of pleasurable activities experienced, and work together to discover how, when, and where to increase pleasurable activity scheduling (also known as *behavioral activation*). Between subsequent sessions, the client will be asked to keep track of his or her efforts to increase pleasurable activities. That information can then be analyzed in-session with the therapist to identify any barriers to participating in pleasurable activities, such as shyness or difficulty with assertiveness.

CBT and Anxiety

Anxiety is another common psychological feature that may be a direct consequence of MS disease progression, a consequence of loss and change related to the disorder, or a combination of both. According to Aaron Beck's schema theory (see Beck & Beck, 2011), mood disorders (anxiety included) arise from and are maintained by unreasonable and maladaptive thoughts. One common CBT treatment for anxiety involves the thought record – an ongoing assessment and intervention of the client's automatic thoughts, the context under

Table 22
Ten Common Maladaptive Thoughts (see Beck & Beck, 2011)

Polarized thinking	The world is perceived in extremes – as either all good or all bad; all positive or all negative.
Personalization	Causation – especially of negative events – is attributed to one's self.
Jumping to conclusions	Making inferences based on incomplete information.
Mind reading	Making inferences about the intentions of others without adequate information.
Control fallacies	The belief that one is responsible for the happiness of others.
Overgeneralization/ filtering	Making inferences based on a single, often negative, occurrence.
Catastrophizing	Overestimating the likeliness of failure based on a single, negative event/occurrence.
Shoulds	The rigid belief in certain ways that one must think, behave, or feel.
Emotional reasoning	Over-reliance on feelings, rather than less subjective forms of evidence.
Fallacy of change	The belief that one can readily influence the feelings, beliefs, or behaviors of others.

which they occur, and their effect on mood and behavior (see Table 22). For example a common thought distortion associated with anxiety is *personalization*, a distortion in which causation – especially for negative events – is attributed to one's self. Another common maladaptive thought process among persons with depression is *catastrophizing*, in which a person believes all efforts will result in a negative outcome. The role of the thought record in anxiety is to help clients and therapists work together to identify distorted thoughts and then to systematically challenge and change them in a process referred to as cognitive restructuring. Once restructured, the maladaptive thoughts are believed to no longer exist to negatively influence the client's mood.

CBT and Chronic Pain

Chronic pain is a common complication of MS. Developed in the mid-1980s, acceptance and commitment therapy (ACT) is a third wave of CBT that emphasizes mindfulness, attention to the present, and a commitment toward wellness. The major goal of ACT is to mitigate the effects of stress. This is especially important with regard to pain, because negative moods (e.g., depression and anxiety) are associated with increased perception of pain and the exacerbation of pain behavior. Overall, ACT appears to have better short- and longer-term effects than no treatment or treatment as usual when treating pain and its psychosocial correlates (Nordin & Rorsman, 2012; Sheppard, Forsyth, Hickling, & Bianchi, 2010; Simpson et al., 2014).

Although promising, criticism of the ACT approach to the mitigation of MS pain includes a lack of consistency of treatment across studies (e.g., ACT appears to be a mixture of approaches), very small sample sizes, inconsistently measured outcomes, and a relative lack of replicated studies.

Medical Family Therapy

McDaniel and coworkers (1992) proposed a biopsychosocial approach to families with health problems, which they termed *medical family therapy*. Although there appears to be no MS-specific research, this model grows out of the large body of literature on the efficacy of family therapy and is now being offered as an area of specialization in several graduate-level programs in the United States. The medical family therapy approach recommends involving the entire family from the beginning. McDaniel and colleagues (1992) based medical family therapy on the tenet that all human problems are biopsychosocial systems problems. They believe "therapeutic issues involve complex system dynamics at biological, psychological, interpersonal, institutional and community levels" (p. 26). This form of therapy invites therapists to develop an understanding of medical cultures and healthcare providers. The goals are to help the family join together to cope with the illness or disability and promote self-determination in the family and the patient.

McDaniel and colleagues highlight Richard Totman's concepts of *agency* and *communion* as the goals of medical family therapy. McDaniel et al. use the term *agency* to describe active involvement in and commitment to one's own care. The therapist can promote agency by helping the client and family to negotiate for more information and better healthcare and make lifestyle changes. In addition, the therapist can assist the client in learning how to set and communicate boundaries and needs for assistance with family members.

The term *communion* refers to the emotional bonds that are frayed by CID and contact with the healthcare system. McDaniel et al. propose that CID can provide an opportunity for resolving old conflicts and forging new levels of healthy bonding. For example, a client whose family role has required being a strong, independent helper can learn to request and receive help from others.

Help seeking and receiving help can enhance family bonding when a client accepts their family's demonstrations of love and support

Disability-Affirmative Therapy

Disability-affirmative therapy has been recognized by the American Psychological Association as a framework for psychotherapy with people with physical disabilities (http://www.apa.org/pubs/videos/4310915.aspx). Developed by Rhoda Olkin (2009), disability-affirmative therapy provides a template of areas to be assessed in treatment that help the clinician neither over-emphasize nor underestimate the role of disability in the presenting problems and case formulation. The goal is on empowerment and acknowledgement of social marginalization and environmental barriers. For a person with MS who identifies as having a disability, disability-affirmative therapy appreciates the dynamic nature of disability, addresses the medical realities of persons with disabilities, and recognizes personal coping strategies.

The hallmarks of disability-affirmative therapy are affirmative goal setting, an integrated view of the self, and the values of flexibility and creativity that are needed to negotiate the environment (Olkin, 2009). Using established therapeutic practices (e.g., CBT, behavioral therapy, relaxation techniques) within a disability-affirmative framework allows for an integrated approach that includes addressing the individual's presenting symptoms as well as facilitating awareness of social and political factors that may be affecting quality of life.

Self-Management Model

Research with CID indicates that the self-management model is effective for increasing self-efficacy, improving health status, and decreasing pain (Meade & Chronin, 2012). Self-management involves education, skill building, problem solving, communication, and relaxation. The role of the therapist is assessment, psychotherapy, education of healthcare providers, developing programs, and advocacy. Research suggests that self-management is strongly associated with *perceived control* and that both perceived control and self-management mediate the impact that MS has on the quality of life (Bishop, Frain, & Tschopp, 2008).

Meade and Chronin (2012) describe the self-management model as incorporating two concepts, expert patient and self-management. *Expert patient* refers to the inherent knowledge that individuals living with CID have about their diagnosis or disability, its impact on their lives, and what decisions they feel comfortable making. It is a term used to acknowledge the role of an individual with CID in managing his or her health and life. *Self-management* refers to the ability of individuals to manage their health and its physical and psychosocial consequences. However, not all clients will have the inclination or ability to assume the role of expert patient or self-manage.

Positive Psychology

The concept of positive psychology was introduced by Seligman and Csikszentmihalyi in 2000 and has grown in its application to rehabilitation psychology (Pakenham, 2012). It recognizes that there is not only an adverse impact of illness but there also can be positive outcomes. Studies of those with MS have documented both the distress of living with the disease and the benefits. This includes the positive outcomes of personal growth, life satisfaction, and increased well-being and incorporates the resilience factors of acceptance, optimism, and benefit-finding (Pakenham, 2012).

4.1.8   Stress Management

Recent research has documented a positive correlation between stress management, coping interventions, and diminishing symptoms. One study examined the hypothesis that coping moderates the relationship between stress and the development of new brain lesions in MS. The findings provide support for the hypothesis that coping can moderate the relationship between stress and MS (Mohr et al., 2012). In a study of 121 people with relapsing MS, a 24-week stress management program reduced disease activity on MRI scans significantly more than in a control group. However, the benefits were not sustained after the program ended, indicating the need for additional research (Mohr et al., 2012).

There is a strong body of research that points to the efficacy of interventions that mitigate stress in the general population. Although some behavioral health practitioners who work with the MS population utilize these interventions, there has been little MS-specific research in this area. These interventions are CBT, mindfulness meditation, hypnosis, imagery, and relaxation techniques. Somatic experiencing and biofeedback have also been shown to mitigate the effects of stress in the general population (Bowling 2007; Phillips and Levine, 2012).

4.1.9   Pain Management

A complete history includes symptoms and severity; pain management methods employed and the client's assessment of their effectiveness; impact on daily routines; and quality of life. The McGill Pain Questionnaire (Melzack, 1975) is a useful tool for both evaluating pain and providing descriptive language for a client. In addition, consulting with the treating physician will allow for more effective medication assessment and monitoring.

Obtaining a full pain history is an essential component of pain management

Treatment

> **Clinical Pearl**
> **Pain Management**
>
> Pain management is a complex process that is best addressed by a multimodal approach. No singular intervention is effective for managing every type of pain, and clinical interventions tend to lose their effectiveness over time. Therefore, many pain management specialists incorporate a number of interventions into treatment.

Kerns, Kassirer et al. (2002) recommend a multidimensional approach to the assessment and management of MS-related pain, guided by a comprehensive biopsychosocial model. Pain management involves:
1. Initial and continuous evaluation of medical interventions.
2. Evaluating and strengthening coping mechanisms.
3. Utilizing psychological interventions.
4. Encouraging physical interventions.
5. Support clients' exploration of safe CAM interventions.

Interventions

Medical/Surgical
Medical management of MS-related chronic pain is complicated because there are no clear guidelines for pharmacological treatment, it has a poor success rate, and pain medications can lose their effectiveness over time (Kerns et al., 2002). Furthermore, pharmacological pain management may inadvertently complicate efforts to manage other symptoms of MS (Kerns et al., 2002). For example, medications for pain can increase fatigue and impair cognitive and motor functioning. Sometimes, surgical intervention will be recommended when medications and other interventions fail. In addition, people whose pain is unmanaged through conventional means, and those who may be experiencing difficult side effects or prefer a nonmedical treatment, may seek CAM interventions.

Behavioral Health Treatment

> **Clinical Pearl**
> **The Roles of Mental Health Professionals**
>
> There are several roles that mental health professionals can serve: (a) increasing a client's accurate communication about pain to physicians (see Appendix 4) and significant others; (b) consultation with the treating physician; (c) increasing psychological adjustment and quality of life and instruction in pain management techniques.

Certain populations may be at greater risk of their pain concerns being minimized by a medical professional, requiring a mental health professional to assist a physician in understanding the magnitude of a client's discomfort. For example, Drwecki, Moore, Ward, and Prkachin (2011) noted that African Americans may receive lower quality pain treatment. An empathy-inducing, perspective-taking intervention led to a reduction in pain treatment bias.

Behavioral Health Interventions

Stress management is an important component of pain management

Cognitive behavioral therapy, psychoeducation, and mind–body interventions have been found to be effective in reducing pain and pain perception. Behavioral health techniques may target the psychological response and/or the physiological response. Additionally, since there is increasing evidence that stress to can lead to increased pain, mental health professionals are more frequently incorporating stress management techniques into pain management.

Pain Acceptance

Acceptance is generally described as having two parts: *pain willingness* and *activity engagement*. Pain willingness refers to being willing to live with pain, to reduce the frustration of attempting to make the pain go away, while continuing to utilize methods that decrease discomfort. Activity engagement reflects the idea of moving on with life, doing the things that matter even though there is pain.

Pain acceptance has been shown to be related to positive adjustment to chronic pain in patients presenting with pain as a primary problem (Kratz, Hirsch, Ehde, & Jensen, 2013). Kratz and coworker's (2013) research of pain acceptance with those diagnosed with neurological disorders documented that activity engagement predicted lower pain interference and depression and

> **Case Vignette**
> **Roger – Pain Management**
>
> Roger is an upper-level manager whose primary presenting problem was MS-related pain. His pain was being managed pharmacologically; however, the side effects of increased fatigue and cognitive difficulties prevented him from being able to fully utilize these medications at work. Although initially reluctant to explore mind–body techniques, Roger became quite proficient at self-hypnosis, imagery, and somatic experiencing. He successfully employed these techniques at his workplace to decrease his perception of pain, which in turn led to both a decrease in pain medication and an increase in functioning.

greater quality of life and social role satisfaction. Pain willingness predicted less pain interference and depression. Table 23 presents a list of interventions for pain.

Table 23
Pain Interventions

Physical	Psychological	CAM
Heat/cold application	CBT	Medical marijuana
Physical therapy and physiotherapy	Biofeedback	Herbs and supplements
Exercise/movement	Hypnosis and imagery	Acupuncture/acupressure
Massage	Mindfulness meditation	Energy therapies
	Progressive relaxation	
	Somatic Experiencing	

4.1.10 Fatigue Management

Fatigue, one of the most common and debilitating MS symptom, has several psychosocial ramifications. Fatigue is hidden and difficult to explain to others; it interferes with work performance, family participation, and socialization; it is unpredictable and, therefore, difficult to plan for. Fatigue can also mimic some depressive symptoms, complicating assessment and treatment. There are documented physiological contributors to MS-related fatigue, and stress, pain, depression, anxiety, poor sleep and diet, and lack of exercise can all increase fatigue. Fortunately, there are medical and behavioral health interventions that target some of these areas.

Educating client about pacing and balance will allow them to optimize their energy. *Pacing* is matching tasks to ability and energy reserves. This includes knowing what part of the day a person has the most energy, breaking tasks down into smaller parts, building in long or short rest periods, and monitoring energy levels and needs for breaks – even during higher-energy periods (see Appendix 3). *Balance* focuses on realistic assessment of abilities and work, family and/or social activities and responsibilities, and finding the balance between what is desirable and what is possible. This includes incorporating assistance at many levels to optimize quality of life.

4.1.11 Mind–Body Interventions

Mind/body therapies have been shown to improve symptoms that affect quality of life in the non-MS population. Preliminary research indicates that mind–body interventions have a positive effect on depression, anxiety, fatigue, quality of life, bladder incontinence, balance, and daily pain intensity in people with MS (Senders, Wahbeh, Spain, & Shinto, 2012). Senders et al. further concluded that these interventions hold strong potential for use with MS clients, because they often have a calming effect on the autonomic nervous system, appear to be safe, and can be utilized in conjunction with conventional treatment, especially when there is psychosocial stress or need for non-pharmacological options.

An interesting side note is that mind–body techniques can have a positive effect on providers as well as clients. In 2008, the Courage Center in Minneapolis trained their rehabilitation staff in mind–body techniques to utilize with their patients. They reported that at the conclusion of the year-long training, significant changes were found in staff job satisfaction, reported quality of life, job stress, and commitment to employer and profession (Flinn & Olson, 2010).

Biofeedback

Monitoring instruments are used to display readouts of a person's bodily functions, such as heart rate and muscle tension. Preliminary research indicates that biofeedback may be beneficial for addressing MS-associated insomnia, anxiety, pain, and incontinence (http://www.neurologycare.net/biofeedback.html).

Guided Imagery

The American Academy of Guided Imagery defines *guided imagery* as a wide variety of techniques, including simple visualization and direct suggestion using imagery, metaphor, and story-telling as well as active imagination. Therapeutic guided imagery allows clients to enter a relaxed state of mind and then to focus their attention on images associated with the issues they are confronting. For example, people coping with chronic pain can be invited to visit and experience an "inner sanctuary" where there is no pain (http://www.academyforguidedimagery.com).

Guided imagery is a technique frequently used in hypnosis as well as in meditation and other relaxation therapies. There is scant MS-specific research, but the effectiveness of guided imagery for pain management and relaxation is well documented (http://www.academyforguidedimagery.com/research/chronic/nerve/). One study with MS found that use of the relaxation/imagery protocol led to clinically significant reductions in state anxiety (Maguire, 1996).

Clinical Pearl
Helping Clients Achieve a Deeper State of Relaxation

Discover, with your client, a comfortable situation. Assist your client to achieve a deeper state of relaxation by sitting or lying down and breathing deeply and easily. Suggest that your client imagine a comfortable situation. For example, floating on water that is the perfect temperature and feeling the body just let go, relax, and become more and more comfortable may be a perfect image. Suggest that as your client imagines this scene, her or his body can become more comfortable in the office.

Hypnosis

The American Society of Clinical Hypnosis (ASCH, n.d.) defines clinical or medical hypnosis as a state of inner absorption, concentration, and focused attention induced by licensed therapists as a method for treating psychological or physical problems. Recent research supports the view that hypnotic communication and suggestions effectively change physiological and neurological functions (http://www.asch.net/Public/GeneralInfoonHypnosis/DefinitionofHypnosis.aspx). When hypnotized, a person may experience physiologic changes, such as a slowing of the pulse and respiration or relaxing a part of the body that is tightening. In this state, a person may become more open to specific suggestions and goals, such as reducing pain or behavioral change Treatment with hypnosis often includes instructing clients in self-hypnosis and providing them with recordings for home practice (Elkins, Jensen, & Patterson, 2007).

Wainapel and Fast (2003) noted that 40 years ago, Baer, Becker, and Wright first wrote about the use of hypnotic interventions to facilitate psychological as well as physical change in rehabilitation. Since then, hypnotic interventions have been successfully utilized to enhance functional ability, decrease pain, mediate emotional responses to disability, decrease spasticity, increase range of motion, increase bowel and bladder control, reeducate movement, and increase motivation (Appel, 1992, 2003). Hypnosis has also been found to decrease stress and inflammation, as well as increase relaxation, comfort, and sleep in the general population.

In studies of other conditions, hypnosis reduced symptoms that also occur commonly in association with MS, such as anxiety, insomnia, and pain. Additionally, hypnosis can help those living with disability to prepare for work by assisting them with job interview performance anxiety and rehearsal of various job tasks. Hypnosis has been associated with improvements in energy and reductions in the emotional and physical difficulties in those with MS (Appel, 2003; http://www.neurologycare.net/hypnosis.html). Before utilizing hypnosis for symptom management, mental health professionals should receive proper training, and clients should be screened for psychological stability.

Hypnosis for Pain

Hypnosis has a long and well-documented history as a pain management tool. In a review of 13 studies, Elkins, Jensen, & Patterson (2007) determined that hypnosis interventions consistently produce significant decreases in pain associated with a variety of chronic pain. Jensen et al. (2005) reported significant improvement in pain intensity, pain unpleasantness, and perceived control over pain in patients with chronic pain secondary to a disability. Jensen, Ende, & Gertz, et al. (2010) described the efficacy of self-hypnosis training for the management of chronic pain in persons with MS. In addition, hypnosis may have other benefits for people with MS, such as reduced anxiety and improved sleep (Bowling, 2007).

Clinical Pearl
Example of a Hypnosis Script for Pain

This hypnotic technique, with practice, can be utilized with the eyes open to bring relief to people in the workplace. In a deep state of relaxation, the client is invited to imagine a dial or dimmer switch with numbers from 1 to 10. Some more technically sophisticated clients may have different images, which are equally effective. Being able to visualize the dimmer is not as important as just imagining that it is there. The client is asked to rate their current level of discomfort and to imagine that the "dial" is set on that number, as the dial directly corresponds to the level of their discomfort. There is then a suggestion that with each breath out the client imagine that the dial is being turned down just a little, resulting in an incremental decrease in discomfort.

Hypnosis for Stress Management

Similar to pain management, hypnosis can be utilized to relax the body and mind, as well as to decrease stress. In a state of relaxation, a different response to a stressor can be rehearsed. Beforehand, review with the client those situations that cause stress, how the client would like to feel and think, and what suggestions would be helpful. In this way, hypnosis can increase self-efficacy.

Case Vignette

Marie – Fear of Stairs

Although Marie had some numbness in her feet, she was physically able to negotiate the stairs in front of her house and had not fallen. However, her anxiety about falling made her reluctant to utilize both the stairs in front of her house and at friends' homes. During hypnosis, each section of going down the steps was rehearsed in her imagination. Each part was accompanied with the suggestion of increasing confidence, stability, and alert relaxation with a focus on feeling her grip on the railing and hearing her feet on the steps. She was also given permission to move at the pace that was most comfortable to her. As Marie did not have difficulty standing from a seated position, when she was holding on to the railing, she was also given the suggestion that she could sit down on a step if she wanted to slow the process down. She practiced it at home first as self-hypnosis, then in vivo. After making it successfully down the stairs a few times, without feeling anxious, she became more willing to engage in activities outside of her home.

Meditation

There are many different types of meditation practices, but all of them seek to promote mental calmness through self-observation of mental activity and cultivating a nonjudgmental attitude that highlights process rather than content. The central element of mindfulness is to remain present in the current moment and practice nonjudgmental acceptance of internal (bodily sensations, breath, thoughts, emotions) and external (sights, sounds) stimuli. Mindfulness meditation has been formalized for clinical interventions with mindfulness-based stress reduction and mindfulness-based cognitive therapy (Wahbeh, Elsas, & Oken, 2008). Developed by Dr. Jon Kabat-Zinn in 1979, mindfulness-based stress reduction (MBSR) has been utilized for stress and pain reduction in both the general and clinical population (Kabat-Zinn, 2011).

As with the general public, meditation can be an effective stress-reduction technique for people living with MS. Grossman et al. (2010) found evidence of improved health-related quality of life and well-being with a program of mindfulness training for persons with MS.

Relaxation and Breathing Techniques

Relaxation and breathing techniques utilize awareness of breathing rate, rhythm, and volume. Most often breathing techniques are used to minimize physiologic responses to stress, possibly by increasing parasympathetic response. Breathing techniques are frequently used in conjunction with relaxation techniques (Wahbeh et al., 2008).

Psychoneuroimmunology

Psychoneuroimmunology examines the interactions between the nervous and immune systems, and the ways in which these interactions affect behavior and health. There is no published research on psychoneuroimmunology and MS. However, we mention it here because there is a connection between stress and MS, and psychoneuroimmunology investigation has highlighted the relationship between stress and its physiological effects on the body (Bowling, 2007). In addition, psychoneuroimmunology techniques, which utilize the placebo effect for pain management, may hold promise for those with MS-related pain.

Somatic Experiencing

Originally developed by Peter Levine to treat trauma, somatic experiencing targets the physiological fight, flight, freeze responses to traumatic memories and employs techniques to calm and nullify them. Although there is no MS-specific research, it is worth mentioning because of anecdotal reports and several publications related to stress and pain relief in the general public (e.g., Phillips, 2007; Phillips & Levine, 2012). Somatic experiencing holds promise as a gentle intervention that, with practice, may be utilized outside of a clinician's office.

4.1.12 Group-Based Interventions

According to the extant literature, group-based interventions are effective and cost-effective treatment modalities for many health-related conditions, including MS (e.g., Humphreys, Drummond, Phillips, & Lincoln, 2013). For the sake of this section, group-based interventions will be defined as treatments offered to sets of three or more individuals with a common concern (e.g., living with a diagnosis of MS, taking care of someone living with MS, etc.). Group-based interventions come in many modalities – from peer-led, self-help groups that focus on emotional support; to professional-led, psychotherapy groups that emphasize behavioral techniques to manage stress; to various combinations of the two. Some group modalities are brief (weekly sessions for 5–15 weeks) and focus strictly on psychoeducation, while others may run indefinitely and aim to systematically change behaviors and worldviews via traditional, psychotherapeutic treatment modalities, including existential/ experiential, psychodynamic, humanistic, and cognitive-behavioral approaches.

For individuals living with MS, group-based interventions – when done well – offer an opportunity to meet with similar others in a supportive, nonjudgmental environment that encourages the acquisition of helpful information and skills, the liberal exchange of social support, and emotional disclosure.

The role of the group leader – either professional or trained peer – is to create and maintain an environment in which self-disclosure and emotional expression can be safely exchanged among group members.

Although the extant literature finds that group-based interventions for MS are better than no treatment or treatment as usual, different modalities may

Meeting other persons who are going through a similar experience can be stigmatizing but also potentially enlightening

not be equally effective for a variety of health-related outcomes (e.g., Mohr et al., 2001). For example, in a small literature comparing the effectiveness of peer-led supportive versus professionally led informational groups for women living with breast cancer, Helgeson and colleagues found that clients gained more information from informational groups, and this effect was long-lasting (Helgeson, Cohen, Schulz, & Yasko, 1999, 2000, 2001). Moreover, Helgeson and colleagues found that emotion-focused peer support groups were associated with greater distress in the short-term (Helgeson et al., 1999). One possible explanation not explored by the investigators was that the study outcomes might have been biased toward favoring the attainment and retention of information – an outcome more likely to be associated with an information-focused therapeutic approach than an emotion-focused one. Similarly, the short-term increase in distress among participants who were enrolled in the support group condition of the study may have been, in actuality, an indication of increased awareness that often occurs in emotion-focused group psycho-therapies. Despite these potential issues, Helgeson's studies make it clear that group-based interventions may not be for everyone all the time.

4.2   Working With Physicians and Other Healthcare Providers

Treatment of MS requires a team approach, with the individual living with MS at the center of that team. Such an approach helps to determine the variety of services and interventions that an individual may need, with the overall goal to improve quality of life. The individual with MS is engaged in decision making with regard to potential short-term and long-term treatment options. These options not only include medications, but also access to rehabilitative specialists (e.g., physical therapy for mobility problems), other medical professionals (e.g., meeting with a urologist to address bladder control problems), and/or psychological resources (e.g., engaging in psychotherapy to address depression). The team approach evolves as the disease progresses and can also depend on the subtype of MS the client is experiencing. As the need arises, bringing in these additional resources can enhance quality of life.

Psychologists working with MS patients may need to consult with other treatment providers, including medical and rehabilitation professionals. Such collaboration among providers can maximally aid the client. An open dialogue, rather than treating in isolation, allows providers to work together for the client's benefit. This also reduces frustration and confusion for the client, who may be getting mixed messages from different providers. Mental health providers may consider suggesting that another specialist be added to the treatment team, which often requires consultation with a neurologist or coordinating medical provider.

It is often important to request a copy of the client's most recent medical chart note, as well as any pertinent consultation reports that the healthcare provider has ordered (e.g., a cognitive evaluation or psychological evaluation). When discussing a mutual client, having a list of concise questions and prioritizing them by matter of importance is often helpful given time constraints.

It is also important to ensure that you have obtained a signed consent from the client and follow guidelines imposed by the Health Insurance Portability and Accountability Act. Informing the healthcare provider of concerns, such as mood disorders, psychosis, or personality disorders, or marked personality changes that are a prominent feature of the clinical picture, is of utmost importance. In particular, treatment-interfering behaviors, such as substance abuse or injection phobia, and/or psychiatric changes that temporally coincide with medical treatment changes should be shared with the medical provider. If psychosocial issues are present, such as limited financial resources or limited academic achievement, it is important to share this information. Similarly, important cultural variables may be helpful to share (e.g., the client's cultural view of their medical provider).

4.3   Efficacy and Prognosis

Treatment decisions balance the benefits of individual interventions with their risks and side effects. Effective treatments have been established that potentially alter the clinical outcomes and disease course of MS. Additional medications with various mechanisms of action await approval pending clinical trials. Currently, clinical trials are being conducted on future medications that aim to repair the CNS in individuals living with MS. With regard to relatively new medications, such as oral disease-modifying treatments, the long-term safety and efficacy are not yet known. Other treatments include cognitive rehabilitative interventions, and it appears that these interventions are effective. That said, work remains in this area, particularly with regard to durability of outcome over long durations of time, as well as determining whether skills can be generalized from specific gains made in treatment to daily living tasks.

4.3.1   Neuropsychological Prognosis

Pharmacologic and nonpharmacologic interventions have been utilized to address cognitive dysfunction. DMT may improve cognitive function through the prevention of new lesions or potentially through the deceleration of neurodegeneration (Julian, 2011). A few rigorous studies have been conducted to address cognitive rehabilitation in MS, with promising results suggested. Specifically, individuals can benefit from training aimed at improving executive functions, learning, and memory. Both structural and functional changes on neuroimaging are related to improvements in cognitive abilities in MS following cognitive rehabilitation. Similarly, some researchers have promoted physical exercise to enhance general health, including cognitive functioning. The impact of aerobic and resistance training programs on cognitive and functional abilities is being studied in MS populations.

4.4   Variations and Combinations of Methods

While there may be documented evidence of a variation or combination of interventions for a specific psychiatric or MS-related symptom, there is no evidence of this for MS in general. However, the NMSS promotes the model of comprehensive, coordinated MS care to address the complexity of the MS disease process (http://www.nationalmssociety.org/Treating-MS/Comprehensive-Care).

In addition, an emerging trend with MS centers is to include professionals from many fields on the treatment team. This is necessary because a combination of modalities and interventions can be more effective than any single treatment.

4.5   Problems in Carrying Out the Treatments

4.5.1   Managing Ambivalence, Conflicts, and Ambiguity

The numerous available treatment choices, and the confusion and frustration that can accompany MS, can become overwhelming for both the client and the professional. In addition, a mental health professional may feel pulled to rescue, advise, or give opinions. However, in this situation, the therapist's role is twofold: She must validate the client's ambivalence, contradictory desires, and beliefs and at the same time provide interventions aimed at lowering anxiety and enabling informed decisions. This process can become particularly challenging when the professional has strong opinions. It is therefore important for a mental health professional to understand personal biases and/or fears around illness and disability, manage personal conflict and ambiguity, and seek psychotherapy or consultation when necessary.

Hope/Denial
It is important for clients to believe that treatment and interventions will help them, but they may have unrealistic expectations and become disappointed. In addition, some clients have so much faith that a cure will be found or a treatment will work that they are not motivated to explore additional options.

Independence/Help Seeking
Some clients base their identity on being independent, strong, and/or a helper. They may need assistance in learning how to ask for and to accept help. For example, some people would rather walk holding on to the wall (wall walking) then use a mobility aid. Conversely, some may undervalue their abilities and become unnecessarily dependent and will need help in becoming more self-reliant.

Chronic Illness/Disability
Those who identify as having a disability may resist the notion that they are "sick." Conversely, those who identify as having a chronic illness may view disability as an indication that their symptoms will progress. Therefore, one person may love the flexibility that a handicapped-parking placard can bring

while for another, the wheelchair symbol hanging from their rear-view mirror elicits apprehension about what the future might hold.

However, with either identity, clients often feel alienated from community support. For example, someone with a hearing impairment, who identifies as a member of the disability community, may not relate to the medical aspect of MS. Similarly, someone with a more consistent mobility challenge may be confused by the fluctuating need to use mobility aids that can exist with MS.

Awareness of Future/Fear of the Future
Although it is important for clients and their families to realistically plan for the possibility that the MS may progress, it is equally important for people to be able enjoy their present lives. For example, a client with MS and no mobility difficulties might be looking for a new home. Some will choose the favorite option, even if there are some stairs, and move if the need arises. Others may choose a less desirable place, but a home without stairs, because the thought of having to possibly move again increases stress.

Disability Benefits
If and when a person should apply for disability benefits are complicated questions. There can be a sense of independence, community, structure, and pride that can come from working, and thus leaving the workforce can affect identity and quality of life. However, if disabilities significantly impair ability to function at work, leaving work can be a great relief and may enable a person to participate more fully in family or community activities.

Frustrations With Healthcare Providers
It is important for a client to trust his or her doctors. Therefore, when a client is distressed because a doctor's office is unresponsive or unsupportive during an exacerbation, it is important to be aware of validating the frustration without undermining confidence. However, if the client wishes to seek another healthcare provider, this decision needs to be supported. In addition, frustration with the logistics, limitations, and expense of healthcare and the lack of treatment alternatives can also influence a client's attitude toward the mental health provider and the therapeutic process.

Medications and Other Medical Interventions
Ultimately, it is up to the client, in consultation with his or her healthcare providers, to decide whether to pursue a treatment or not. This becomes more complicated when a treatment is either causing or has the potential to cause uncomfortable side effects, is experimental, or it is unclear if the proposed treatment will be effective for the client. Clients may be indecisive, scared, and confused and need to feel that therapy is a safe place to explore all options. Therapist bias can interfere in this process.

Flexibility/Boundaries
Providers need to flexible. For example, symptom flares or logistics may prevent a client from coming for a session and the client may cancel with short notice. It is important to plan for this in the initial session. This may include substituting

phone sessions, allowing for a rescheduled visit without penalty, or home visits. However, therapist boundaries need to be considered in this negotiation.

Clients may also need additional considerations; For example, clients who use a wheelchair or scooter may need assistance transferring to a chair or a chair that is easy to rise from. Clients may also need a change in temperature or lighting. However, a client may be ashamed to ask or be offended by a therapist's offer of assistance. Again, this can be discussed either in the first session or prior to it: "I want my clients to feel as comfortable as possible in my office so, let's talk about your needs. Are you sensitive to heat or light, or do you need assistance transferring?"

4.5.2   Medical Interventions

Once scant, the advent of disease-modifying therapies and adjunctive treatments for symptom management has made treatment-related decision making overwhelming for many individuals. The desire to select the most effective interventions when offered multiple options can exacerbate a client's distress. Likewise, anxious avoidance may pose as a barrier to engaging in a needs assessment (e.g., evaluating the benefit of assistive devices, evaluating the benefit of prescribed physical therapy exercises to reduce fall risk, evaluating the benefit of cognitive rehabilitation). Patti (2010) identified various factors that impact engagement in medical treatment:

1. Disease- and treatment-related issues to adherence
   - Access to information about MS and treatment options
   - Adverse side effects and/or injection site reactions
   - Convenience of dosing (autoinjector)
   - Utilization of self-injection training
   - Individual receives care at an MS care center or specialty center, or by specialty provider
   - Stable disease, lack of symptoms; belief that treatment is not necessary
   - Doubt about the diagnosis
   - Cannot afford treatment
   - Pregnancy
2. Mental health- and neuropsychological-related issues to adherence
   - Depression, anxiety, perceived lack of self-efficacy
   - Avoidance, fear of bringing the disease to mind on a regular basis by engaging in treatments
   - Needle/injection phobia
   - Substance abuse or dependence
   - Cognitive dysfunction
   - Emotionally drained, no longer motivated to engage in treatment

4.5.3   Noncompliance/Resistance

It is important to view a client with MS through both a mental and physical health lens. This means that what appears to be resistance, for example, could be indicative of a cognitive or fatigue-related difficulty. Similarly, if MS symptoms wax and wane, the client may change in demeanor; sometimes presenting as engaging, insight-oriented, independent, or optimistic; at other times appearing inattentive, negative, or dependent. Although these behavioral shifts may be indicative of insubstantial coping skills and psychiatric diagnoses, they can also be the consequence of fatigue and/or navigation with painful or debilitating symptoms.

4.6   Multicultural Issues

An individual's multicultural context can influence all aspects of health, including health beliefs (e.g., disease etiology) and health behaviors (e.g., symptom expression, sources of social support).

Most individuals simply consider issues related to race, culture, or ethnicity when it comes to multicultural diversity. The scope of diversity, however, is much broader and includes demographic factors such as gender, sexuality, religion, education, social class, and age. Each of these can influence – directly or indirectly, alone or in myriad combinations – how one experiences MS.

Adequately assessing the proximal role that religion may play in a client's life, for example, may give a better understanding as to whether a diagnosis of MS may be perceived as a curse or a challenge (e.g., Pargament, 1997). Religion may also inform who may be an appropriate source of social support (e.g., a rabbi or a minister) or how best to cope.

Not every demographic factor will have an equal influence on health beliefs or health behaviors. Sexual orientation, for example, may play an important role in identifying who may be an important source of social support (e.g., a same-sex partner), but it might not have much of an influence on medical adherence. Alternatively, a client's gender may play a major role in the expression of MS symptoms (e.g., pain behavior), but gender may not tell us much about potentially important differences in understanding disease progression.

The counseling literature has several acronyms that help providers remember the demographic/ecological units that comprise multicultural diversity. One example is Ivey, Ivey, and Zalaquett's (2009) *RESPECTFUL*: **r**eligion/spirituality, **e**conomic/class background, **s**exual identity, **p**ersonal style/education, **e**thnic/racial identity, **c**hronological/lifespan, **t**rauma, **f**amily background, **u**nique physical characteristics, and **l**ocation of residence and language. Hays's (2011) *ADDRESSING* framework also enables mental health workers to better understand cultural influences as a multidimensional combination of ecological units (see Table 24).

An added benefit to Hays's framework is that it allows the mental health worker to assess the social status (minority or majority) of each ecological unit with which a client identifies, giving the added dimensions of power and privilege to the context of the client's MS experience.

It is essential to note that the importance of these factors may change with context and over time. So, for example, while religion for some individuals may not be a salient factor every day, it may certainly become imminently important after a diagnosis of MS or when new symptoms emerge. In addition,

Table 24
Hays's (2011) ADDRESSING Framework

A	Age and generational influences
DD	Developmental and acquired disabilities
R	Religion
E	Ethnic and racial identity
S	Socioeconomic status
S	Sexual orientation
I	Indigenous heritage
N	National origin
G	Gender

ecological units may conflict with one another to challenge a client's quality of life (e.g., a gay, Christian Republican living in the southern United States), or they may work together as a source of pride and strength.

Understanding a client's multicultural identity will help you understand how he or she may be experiencing MS

The role of culture is just beginning to be recognized as an important part of evidence-based treatments for CIDs like MS. There are a number of socio-cultural reasons why individuals of social minority status traditionally have not been included in biomedical or psychological treatment research, and the contexts under which various populations may experience MS, for example, have gone uninvestigated.

However, the fact that something has not been studied does not negate its importance or existence. There is a growing body of sociocultural research and practice-informed knowledge to indicate the importance of multicultural issues in understanding the true impact of MS. As we wait for research evidence to support the importance of multicultural diversity in the treatment of MS, it is important to not throw out the baby with the bath water.

5

Case Vignettes

5.1   Case Vignette: Michelle

Michelle, a Caucasian woman in her mid-20s and newly diagnosed with relapsing–remitting MS, was referred from her neurologist for anxiety and depression. Her primary MS symptom was fatigue. She denied depression prior to diagnosis but endorsed a history of anxiety. She described a tumultuous childhood but there was no history of abuse. Although Michelle was attractive and intelligent, she reported low self-esteem related to her appearance and abilities, and MS accentuated these concerns. Michelle wanted to both pursue a career and get married, and she was afraid that MS would prevent her from reaching these goals. Michelle's therapy was long-term, and she saw her therapist on a regular basis for several years.

Although Michelle denied suicidality, she was crying daily and was pessimistic about the future. She reported having a good relationship with her neurologist and minimal difficulty tolerating the prescribed medication, but she was reluctant to take additional medication for depression. After consultation with Michelle's neurologist, he reframed her depression as a side effect of her MS mediation and strongly recommended a 6-month trial with antidepressants. The medication was very effective in elevating her mood and returning her to what she called "my pre-MS self."

Michelle had educated herself about MS from a medical standpoint, but she did not understand the emotional aspects or the role of self-care in managing symptoms. Once she understood the relationship between psychological stress, her physical stress reaction, and some of her MS symptoms, Michelle was eager to discover ways to intervene. She explained that knowing that there were things that she could do that might make living with MS easier made her feel less powerless.

Initially, psychoeducation about fatigue management, the fight/flight/freeze response, and the role of exercise and sleep hygiene in managing anxiety, stress, and fatigue was introduced. Several stress reduction techniques were then offered to see which was most effective. Clients with a long history of anxiety often believe that their anxiety cannot be treated. It was therefore important for treatment to be framed as a failure-proof experiment and a way to discover together which stress and anxiety management interventions worked best for her. For Michelle, the best results were obtained with the simplest mindfulness, breathing, and somatic experiencing techniques. A recording was made of some of these exercises for her to use at home.

When Michelle felt confident that she had some tools to mitigate her anxiety reactions, she was ready to explore childhood issues, which led to further stability. Michelle learned to realistically evaluate her energy levels and to decrease her anxiety reaction to flare-ups of MS symptoms. Eventually, she was able to manage her anxiety, stress, and MS symptoms well enough to successfully pursue a career. She began to feel more comfortable about dating and discussing her diagnosis with friends. In addition, she found enjoyable ways to exercise, which both decreased her stress and improved her stamina.

5.2   Case Vignette: Claudette

Claudette, an African American woman in her 50s, was newly diagnosed with secondary progressive MS. She had been living with MS symptoms, undiagnosed, for many years and the diagnosis actually brought relief. Her primary symptoms were fatigue and urge incontinence. Although not always the case, for this client, short-term, solution-focused, telephonic therapy was both appropriate and successful.

Claudette's main concerns were her family's difficulty in accepting her diagnosis and her increasing inability to meet her family's needs. Being a good mother and supporting others was an important part of Claudette's identity and cultural values. She had successfully juggled working and parenting when her children were younger and, as she was now retired, she was frustrated that she struggled daily to accomplish what she considered small household chores. Claudette was accustomed to being responsible for all household maintenance and daily upkeep and providing childcare for her grandchildren several days a week. Both her daughter and husband were reluctant to talk to her or others about MS, and because of this she kept her diagnosis from most of her church community.

Therapy initially focused on assessing Claudette's functioning level, coping skills, understanding of MS, and her family concerns. Claudette said that she felt confident in her neurologist's abilities. An assessment of her coping skills indicated that she had dealt well with past difficulties, and she felt that she was coping much better with her diagnosis than the rest of her family.

The following sessions focused on self-care. Claudette had based her identity on helping others and was reluctant to focus on herself. When the situation was framed as the best thing that she could do to help her family was to help herself, she agreed. She and her therapist explored her experience with MS, her feelings about the diagnosis, and fatigue management. She was encouraged to contact the MS Society about a self-help group.

After several sessions, Claudette reported that she attended a support group with her son. She said that just learning about others' experiences helped them both feel better. Her son volunteered to talk with Claudette's husband and daughter about MS and her changing abilities.

However, Claudette wanted her husband to get more involved and struggled with how to get him to participate in an MS Society-sponsored social activity. In the sixth session, she reported that they both attended the event. This led to some realistic but optimistic discussions between them about both their current situation and their future. Having regained her family support, Claudette then shared her diagnosis with her church community and was surprised by the additional support that she received. A short while later, Claudette was ready to terminate therapy.

5.3   Case Vignette: Jon

Jon, a man in his mid-30s, was diagnosed with primary progressive MS 4 months before beginning therapy. He was in good physical shape prior to his diagnosis and continued to exercise but was beginning to notice increasing weakness. Jon reported that he struggled with word finding when he was fatigued but denied other cognitive difficulties. Since Jon's job required superior cognitive functioning, this was a major concern.

Jon was in the United States on a work visa and was striving to become a citizen. He had recently been commended for his exceptional job performance, and his MS symptoms had not affected his ability to work. However, he was afraid of losing his job because of his MS diagnosis, and he had not disclosed his diagnosis at work. He entered therapy to better understand MS and how to manage his symptoms. Jon remained in therapy for 18 months, moving gradually from weekly to monthly sessions.

Jon reported that he had a supportive relationship and friends and no prior history of physical or mental health issues. Fatigue, stress, and pain management were the focus of therapy. Jon was reluctant to use pain medication at work because of side effects, so he was often uncomfortable. Jon responded well to mind–body interventions, including hypnosis, imagery, and somatic experiencing. Recordings were made for him to practice at home, and he quickly learned to use the techniques at work without the recordings.

Most of Jon's stress was work-related and as he became better able to manage his stress, he began to engage more with his coworkers, which in turn alleviated his stress. Jon also became proficient enough in using mind–body techniques that he was able to significantly decrease the discomfort he felt at work, which improved his performance. Eventually, this led to disclosure about his diagnosis to his supervisor, and his boss assured him that he would do whatever he could to keep Jon at his job.

5.4   Case Vignette (Neuropsychological Evaluation): Cassie

Cassie, a 45-year-old female, was referred by her neurologist for a neuropsychological evaluation. She was diagnosed with RRMS 3 years prior. In our work together, Cassie noted that her primary concerns included MS-related fatigue, cognitive problems, depression, and difficulties at work. She and her husband described frequent arguments and feelings of isolation in their marriage.

After the evaluation Cassie and her husband were provided with the results, which revealed weaknesses in processing speed, attention, and memory retrieval. Overall, such difficulties were impacting the quality of her work performance, as well as communication and productivity at home and work. Given the results, Cassie engaged in cognitive rehabilitation sessions focused on learning compensatory strategies. She was also provided with written information on specific work-place modifications to share with her employer, as well as potentially helpful community resources. She learned fatigue management strategies from a MS nurse specialist.

A reciprocal relationship often exists wherein cognitive problems are magnified by mood disturbance. Cassie's depression improved with medication prescribed by her neurologist, engagement in individual counseling, and regular attendance in a NMSS sponsored support group. A lift in her depression coincided with improved use of the cognitive techniques that she was taught.

Her husband's assumption that she was losing interest in their marriage was reframed in light of Cassie's neurocognitive profile. He was relieved when hearing how weaknesses in these areas often translate into problems sustaining attention during conversations and what they could do to bolster communication. They appeared engaged during a collaborative conversation about the impact of MS upon their marriage, which served to normalize their reactions to living with MS; they were validated by hearing that while some couples can draw closer together in mutual support, many couples experience some grief, identity struggles, anxiety, anger, and sadness. They agreed that the ebb and flow of these emotions can take a toll on even the most secure couples. A referral to a marriage and family therapist was initiated. They were encouraged to attend a couple's retreat weekend sponsored by the organization "Can Do Multiple Sclerosis."

6

Further Reading

American Psychological Association. (2001). *An educational pamphlet brought to you by the Public Interest Advisory Committee, Division 40 (Clinical Neuropsychology)*. Washington, DC: Author.

An educational pamphlet that provides information regarding Clinical Neuropsychology, the typical reasons for referral to a neuropsychologist, what clients should expect from engaging in an evaluation, and how the results may be potentially helpful to clients, families, and clinicians.

Beck, J. S., & Beck, A. T. (2011). *Cognitive behavioral therapy: Basics and beyond*. New York, NY: Guilford Publications.

This is a seminal text on the practice of Cognitive Behavioral Therapy.

Burns, D. D. (2008). *Feeling good: The new mood therapy*. New York, NY: New American Library.

This is a popular text for professionals and laypeople alike on the links between mood, thoughts, and behavior.

Carney, C., & Manber, R. (2009). *Quiet your mind & get to sleep: Solutions to insomnia for those with depression, anxiety, or chronic pain*. Oakland, CA: New Harbinger Publications.

A psychoeducational workbook that uses cognitive behavior therapy to address sleep problems in individuals who experience anxiety, depression, and chronic pain. The authors focus on ways to optimize sleep patterns by using methods to calm the mind and to help clients identify sleep-depriving behaviors.

National Multiple Sclerosis Society. (2011). *Depression & multiple sclerosis managing specific issues*. Retrieved from http://www.nationalmssociety.org/NationalMSSociety/media/MSNationalFiles/Brochures/Brochure-Depression.pdf

A psychoeducational brochure that can be shared with clients to engage in dialogue regarding management of depression symptoms in MS.

Olkin, R. (1999). *What psychotherapists should know about disability*. New York, NY: Guilford.

This comprehensive book provides pertinent education to therapists about disability. This, in turn, enables therapists to educate and better support their clients.

Reitman, N., & Kalb, R. (2012). *Multiple sclerosis: A model of psychosocial support* (5th ed.) New York, NY: NMSS Professional Resource Center.

Published by the NMSS and authored by two noted experts in MS, this valuable publication provides a guide to healthy psychosocial adaptation with MS.

Taber, K. H., Hurley, R. A., & Yudofsky, S. C. (2010). Diagnosis and treatment of neuropsychiatric disorders. *Annual Review of Medicine, 61*, 121–133.

The authors provide a review of the most prevalent neuropsychiatric disorders and symptoms present in neurologic populations, as well as a well-informed discussion of psychotropic interventions.

Complementary and Alternative Medicine and Mind–Body Interventions

http://www.mscenter.org/education/complementary-care

www.neurologycare.net

These are two comprehensive websites about MS and CAM interventions.

Hypnosis
http://www.asch.net
Extensive information about hypnosis is provided on the American Association of Clinical Hypnosis website.

Information About MS
National Multiple Sclerosis Society – http://www.nationalmssociety.org
The Consortium of Multiple Sclerosis Centers – http://www.mscare.org/
Can Do Multiple Sclerosis – http://www.mscando.org/
The NMSS maintains an extensive and current website about every aspect of MS; treatments, research, resources and education. It provides access to free information and publications for both professionals and persons living with MS.

7

References

Academy for Guided Imagery. (2006, September). *Using guided imagery for nerve pain – research findings.* Retrieved from http://academyforguidedimagery.com/research/chronic/nerve

Academy for Guided Imagery. (n.d.). *About guided imagery.* Retrieved from http://acadgi.com/abouttheacademy/aboutguidedimagery/index.html

Allen, J. G. (2003). Coping with traumatic stress. *California Psychologist, 36*(1), 16–18.

American Psychiatric Association. (2013). *Diagnostic and statistical manual of mental disorders* (5th ed.). Arlington, VA: Author.

American Psychological Association. (n.d.). *Join the Rehabilitation Psychology Division.* Retrieved from http://www.apadivisions.org/division-22/membership/index.aspx

American Society of Clinical Hypnosis. (n.d.) *Definition of hypnosis.* Retrieved from http://www.asch.net/Public/GeneralInfoonHypnosis/DefinitionofHypnosis.aspx

Appel, P. (2003). Clinical hypnosis in rehabilitation. *Seminars in Integrative Medicine, 1*(2), 90–105. http://doi.org/10.1016/S1543-1150(03)00010-3

Appel, P. R. (1992). The use of hypnosis in physical medicine and rehabilitation. *Psychological Medicine, 10,* 133–148.

Arciniegas, D. B. (2005). A clinical overview of pseudobulbar affect. *The American Journal of Geriatric Pharmacotherapy, 3,* 4–8. http://doi.org/10.1016/S1543-5946(05)80031-5

Askey-Jones, S., David, A. S., Silber, E., Shaw, P., & Chalder, T. (2013). Cognitive behavioral therapy for common mental disorders in people with multiple sclerosis: A benchmark study. *Behavior Research and Therapy, 5,* 648–655. http://doi.org/10.1016/j.brat.2013.04.001

Bandura, A. (1997). *Self-efficacy: The exercise of control.* New York, NY: McMillan.

Beck, A. T., Steer, R. A., & Brown, G. K. (2000). *BDI-Fast screen for medical patients: Manual.* San Antonio, TX: Psychological Corporation.

Beck, J. S., & Beck, A. T. (2011). *Cognitive behavioral therapy: Basics and beyond.* New York. NY: Guilford Publications.

Benedict, R. H., Fischer, J. S., Archibald, C. J., Arnett, P. A., Beatty, W. W., Bobholz, J., ... Munschauer, F. (2002). Minimal neuropsychological assessment of MS patients: A consensus approach. *The Clinical Neuropsychologist, 16*(3), 381–397. http://doi.org/10.1076/clin.16.3.381.13859

Benedict, R. H., Fishman, I., McClellan, M. M., Bakshi, R., & Weinstock-Guttman, B. (2003). Validity of the Beck depression inventory-fast screen in multiple sclerosis. *Multiple Sclerosis, 9*(4), 393–396. http://doi.org/10.1191/1352458503ms902oa

Bishop, M., Frain, M. P., & Tschopp, M. K. (2008). Self-management, perceived control, and subjective quality of life in multiple sclerosis: An exploratory study. *Rehabilitation Counseling Bulletin, 52*(1), 45–56. http://doi.org/10.1177/0034355208320000

Black, P. H. (2002). Stress and the inflammatory response: A review of neurogenic inflammation. *Brain Behavior and Immunity, 16*(6), 622–653. http://doi.org/10.1016/S0889-1591(02)00021-1

Bonanno, G. A., & Mancini, A. D. (2008). The human capacity to thrive in the face of potential trauma. *Pediatrics, 121*(2), 369–375. http://doi.org/10.1542/peds.2007-1648

Bowling, A. (2007). *Complementary and alternative medicine and multiple sclerosis (2nd ed.).* New York, NY: Demos Publishing.

Bowling, N. & Bowling, A. (n.d.). *Lifestyle and alternative medicine.* Retrieved from http://www.neurologycare.net/cam.

Calabrese, M., Bernardi, V., Atzori, M., Mattisi, I., Favaretto, A., Rinaldi, F., ... Gallo, P. (2012). Effect of disease-modifying drugs on cortical lesions and atrophy in relapsing–remitting multiple sclerosis. *Multiple Sclerosis Journal, 18*(4), 418–424. http://doi.org/10.1177/1352458510394702

Caminero, A., & Bartolomé, M. (2011). Sleep disturbances in multiple sclerosis. *Journal of Neurological Sciences, 309*(1–2), 86–91. http://doi.org/10.1016/j.jns.2011.07.015

Carver, C. S., Scheier, M. F., & Weintraub, J.K. (1989). Assessing coping strategies: A theoretically based approach. *Journal of Personality and Social Psychology, 56*(2), 267–283. http://doi.org/10.1037/0022-3514.56.2.267

Castro-Sánchez, A. M., Matarán-Peñarrocha, G., ILara-Palomo, I., Saavedra-Hernández, M., Arroyo-Morales, M., & Moreno-Lorenzo, C. (2012). Hydrotherapy for the treatment of pain in people with multiple sclerosis: A randomized controlled trial, *Evidence-Based Complementary and Alternative Medicine,* 2012, Article ID 473963, 8 pp. http://doi.org/10.1155/2012/473963

Christodoulou, C., Melville, P., Scherl, W. F., Macallister, W. S., Abensur, R. L., Troxell, R. M., & Krupp, L. B. (2009). Negative affect predicts subsequent cognitive change in multiple sclerosis. *Journal of the International Neuropsychological Society, 15*(01), 53–61. http://doi.org/10.1017/S135561770809005X

Chwastiak, L., & Ehde, D. M. (2007). Psychiatric issues in multiple sclerosis. *Psychiatric Clinics of North America, 30*(4), 803–817.

Clark, R., Anderson, N. B., Clark, V. R., & Williams, D. R. (1999). Racism as stressor for African Americans: A biopsychosocial model. *American Psychologist, 54*(10), 805–816. http://doi.org/10.1037/0003-066X.54.10.805

Cohen, S., Janicki-Deverts, D., Doyle, W., Miller, G., Frank, E., Rabin, B. & Turner, R. (2012). Chronic stress, glucocorticoid receptor resistance, inflammation, and disease risk. *Proceedings of the National Academy of Sciences of the United States of America, 109*(16), 5995–5999. http://doi.org/ 10.1073/pnas.1118355109

Comi, G., Martinelli, V., Rodegher, M., Moiola, L., Bajenaru, O., Carra, A., & Filippi, M. (2009). Effect of glatiramer acetate on conversion to clinically definite multiple sclerosis in patients with clinically isolated syndrome (PreCISe study): A randomised, double-blind, placebo-controlled trial. *The Lancet, 374*, 1503–1511. http://doi.org/10.1016/S0140-6736(09)61259-9

Corbin, J. M., & Strauss, A. (1988). *Unending work and care: Managing chronic illness at home.* San Francisco, CA: Jossey-Bass.

Coyle, P. K. (2014). Multiple sclerosis in pregnancy. *CONTINUUM: Lifelong Learning in Neurology, 20*(1), 42–59. http://doi.org/10.1212/01.CON.0000443836.18131.c9

Cree, B. A. (2014). 2014 multiple sclerosis therapeutic update. *The Neurohospitalist, 4*(2), 63–65. http://doi.org/10.1177/1941874414525410

Craig, A. (2012). Resilience in people with disabilities. In P. Kennedy (Ed.), *The Oxford handbook of rehabilitation psychology* (pp. 211–234). New York, NY: Oxford Press.

Damasceno, A., Von Glehn, F., Brandão, C. O., Damasceno, B. P., & Cendes, F. (2013). Prognostic indicators for long-term disability in multiple sclerosis patients. *Journal of the Neurological Sciences, 324*(1), 29–33. http://doi.org/10.1016/j.jns.2012.09.020

Demaree, H., Gaudino, E., & DeLuca, J. (2003). The relationship between depressive symptoms and cognitive dysfunction in multiple sclerosis. *Cognitive Neuropsychiatry, 8*(3), 161–171. http://doi.org/10.1080/13546800244000265

Dennison, L., & Moss-Morris, R. (2010). Cognitive behavioural therapy: What benefits can it offer people with multiple sclerosis? *Expert Review of Neurotherapeutics, s10*(9), 1383–1390. http://doi.org/10.1586/ern.10.111

Dennison, L., Moss-Morris, R., & Chalder, T. (2009). A review of psychological correlates of adjustment in patients with multiple sclerosis. *Clinical Psychology Review, 29*(2), 141–153. http://doi.org/10.1016/j.cpr.2008.12.001

Diaz-Olavarrieta, C., Cummings, J. L., Velazquez, J., & Garcia de la Cadena, C. (1999). Neuropsychiatric manifestations of multiple sclerosis. *Journal of Neuropsychiatry and Clinical Neuroscience, 1*, 51–57. Retrieved from http://www.ncbi.nlm.nih.gov/pubmed/9990556

Drwecki, B., Moore, C., Ward, S., & Prkachin, K. (2011). Reducing racial disparities in pain treatment: The role of empathy and perspective-taking. *PAIN, 15*(2), 1001–1006. http://doi.org/10.1016/j.pain.2010.12.005

Elkins, G., Jensen, M., & Patterson, D. (2007). Hypnotherapy for the management of chronic pain. *International Journal of Clinical Experimental Hypnosis, 55*(3), 275–287. http://doi.org/10.1080/00207140701338621

Falvo, D. (2009). *Medical and psychosocial aspects of chronic illness and disability* (*4th ed.*). Sudbury, MA: Jones and Bartlett.

Feinstein, A., du Boulay, G., & Ron, M. A. (1992). Psychotic illness in multiple sclerosis. A clinical and magnetic resonance imaging study. *The British Journal of Psychiatry, 161*(5), 680–685. http://doi.org/10.1192/bjp.161.5.680

Feinstein, A. (2002). An examination of suicidal intent in patients with multiple sclerosis. *Neurology, 59*(5), 674–678. http://doi.org/10.1212/WNL.59.5.674

Field, B., & Swarm, R. (2008). *Chronic pain*. Cambridge, MA: Hogrefe and Huber.

Figley, C. R. (Ed.) (1995). *Compassion fatigue: Coping with secondary traumatic stress disorder in those who treat the traumatized*. New York, NY: Brunner/Mazel.

Flinn, N., & Olsen, J. (2010). *Mind body integration training: Effects on staff of a rehabilitation facility*. Retrieved from http://www.couragecenter.org/ContentPages/recentresearch.aspx

Forsythe, C. J., & Compas, B. (1987). Interaction of cognitive appraisals of stressful events and coping: Testing the goodness of fit hypothesis. *Cognitive Therapy and Research, 11*(4), 473–485. http://doi.org/10.1007/BF01175357

Fragoso, Y. D., Adoni, T., Anacleto, A., da Gama, P. D., Goncalves, M. V. M., da Cunha Matta, A. P., & Parolin, M. F. K. (2014). Recommendations on diagnosis and treatment of depression in patients with multiple sclerosis. *Practical Neurology, 14*(4), 206–209. http://doi.org/10.1136/practneurol-2013-000735

Frederick, C., & McNeal, S. (1999). *Inner strengths: Contemporary psychotherapy and hypnosis for ego strengthening*. Mahwah, NJ: Erlbaum.

Gadoth, N. (2003). Multiple sclerosis in children. *Brain and Development, 25*(4), 229–232. http://doi.org/10.1016/S0387-7604(03)00035-4

Galetta, S. L., Markowitz, C., & Lee, A. G. (2002). Immunomodulatory agents for the treatment of relapsing multiple sclerosis: A systematic review. *Archives of Internal Medicine, 162*(19), 2161–2169. http://doi.org/10.1001/archinte.162.19.2161

Gaudino, E. A., Chiaravalloti, N. D., DeLuca, J., & Diamond, B. J. (2001). A comparison of memory performance in relapsing-remitting, primary progressive and secondary progressive, multiple sclerosis. *Neuropsychiatry, Neuropsychology, and Behavioral Neurology, 14*(1), 32–44.

Ghaffar, O., & Feinstein, A. (2007). The neuropsychiatry of multiple sclerosis: A review of recent developments. *Current Opinion in Psychiatry, 20*(3), 278–285.

Grossman, P., Kappos, L., Gensicke, M., D'Souza, M., Mohr, D., Penner, I., & Steiner, C. (2010). MS quality of life, depression, and fatigue improve after mindfulness training: A randomized trial. *Neurology, 75*(13), 1141–1149. http://doi.org/10.1212/WNL.0b013e3181f4d80d

Hays, P. A. (2011). *Addressing cultural complexities in practice: Assessment, diagnosis, and therapy* (2nd ed.). Washington, DC: American Psychological Association. http://doi.org/10.1037/11650-000

Heesen, C., Köpke, S., Kasper, J., Poettgen, J., Tallner, A., Mohr, D. C., & Gold, S. M. (2012). Behavioral interventions in multiple sclerosis: a biopsychosocial perspective. *Expert Review of Neurotherapeutics, 12*(9), 1089-1100. http://doi.org/10.1586/ern.12.103

Helgeson, V. S., Cohen, S., Schulz, R., & Yasko, J. (1999). *Education and peer discussion group interventions and adjustment to breast cancer. Archives of General Psychiatry, 56*, 340–347.

Helgeson, V. S., Cohen, S., Schulz, R., & Yasko, J. (2000). Group support interventions for women with breast cancer: Who benefits from what? *Health Psychology, 19*(2), 107–114. http://doi.org/10.1037/0278-6133.19.2.107

Helgeson, V. S., Cohen, S., Schulz, R., & Yasko, J. (2001). *Long-term effects of educational and peer discussion group interventions on adjustment to breast cancer. Health Psychology, 20*(5), 387–392.

Humphreys, I., Drummond, A. E. R., Phillips, C., & Lincoln, N. B. (2013). Cost-effectiveness of an adjustment group for people with multiple sclerosis and low mood: A randomized trial. *Clinical Rehabilitation, 27*(11), 963–971. http://doi.org/10.1177/0269215513488608

Inaloo, S., & Haghbin, S. (2013). Multiple sclerosis in children. *Iranian Journal of Child Neurology, 7*(2), 1–10.

Itkowitz, A., Kerns, R. D., & Otis, J. D. (2003). Support and coronary heart disease. *Journal of Behavioral Medicine, 26*(1), 19–30. http://doi.org/10.1023/A:1021790921471

Ivey, A. E., Ivey, M. B., & Zalaquett, C. P. (2009). *Intentional interviewing and counseling: Facilitating client development in a multicultural society* (7th ed.). Stamford, CT: Cengage Learning.

Janssens, A. C. J. W., Doorn, P. A., Boer, J. B., Meche, F. G. A., Passchier, J., & Hintzen, R. Q. (2003). Impact of recently diagnosed multiple sclerosis on quality of life, anxiety, depression and distress of patients and partners. *Acta Neurologica Scandinavica, 108*(6), 389–395. http://doi.org/10.1034/j.1600-0404.2003.00166.x

Jensen, M. P., Ehde, D. M., Gertz, K. J., Stoelb, B. L., Dillworth, T. M., Hirsh, A. T., … Kraft, G. H. (2011). Effects of self-hypnosis training and cognitive restructuring on daily pain intensity and catastrophizing in individuals with multiple sclerosis and chronic pain. *International Journal of Clinical and Experimental Hypnosis, 59*(1), 45–63. http://doi.org/10.1080/00207144.2011.522892

Jensen, M. P., Hanley, M. A., Engel, J. M., Romano, J. M., Barber, J. B., Cardenas, D. D., … Patterson, D. R. (2005). Hypnotic analgesia for chronic pain in persons with disabilities: A case series. *International Journal of Clinical and Experimental Hypnosis, 53*(2), 198–228. http://doi.org/10.1080/00207140590927545

Jensen, M. P., Molton, I. R., & Kraft, G. H. (2009). Self-hypnosis training for chronic pain management in individuals with multiple sclerosis: Long-term effects. *Multiple Sclerosis, 15*(9), 257. Retrieved from http://msrrtc.washington.edu/node/114

Jensen, M., Barber, J., Romano, J., Molton, I. Raichie, K., Osborne, T., … Patterson, D. (2009). A comparison of self-hypnosis versus progressive muscle relaxation in patients with multiple sclerosis and chronic pain. *International Journal of Clinical and Experimental Hypnosis, 57*(2), 198–221. http://doi.org/10.1080/00207140802665476

Johnson, S. K. (2007). The neuropsychology of multiple sclerosis. *Disease-a-Month, 53*(3), 172–176. http://doi.org/10.1016/j.disamonth.2007.04.009

Jones, S. M., & Amtmann, D. (2014). Health care worry is associated with worse outcomes in multiple sclerosis. *Rehabilitation Psychology, 59*(3), 354. http://doi.org/10.1037/a0037074

Julian, L., Merluzzi, N. M., & Mohr, D. C. (2007). The relationship among depression, subjective cognitive impairment, and neuropsychological performance in multiple sclerosis. *Multiple Sclerosis, 13*(1), 81–86. http://doi.org/10.1177/1352458506070255

Julian, L. J. (2011). Cognitive functioning in multiple sclerosis. *Neurologic Clinics, 29*(2), 507–525. http://doi.org/10.1016/j.ncl.2010.12.003

Kabat-Zinn, J. (1990). *Full catastrophe living: Using the wisdom of your body and mind to face stress, pain, and illness.* New York, NY: Bantam Dell.

Kabat-Zinn, J. (2011). *Mindfulness for beginners: Reclaiming the present moment – and your life.* Boulder, CO: Sounds True.

Kalb, R., Holland, N., & Giesser, B. (2007). *Multiple sclerosis for dummies.* Hoboken, NJ: John Wiley & Sons.

Kalb, R. (2007). The emotional and psychological impact of multiple sclerosis relapses. *Journal of the Neurological Sciences, 256*, S29–S33. http://doi.org/10.1016/j.jns.2007.01.061

Kalb, R. (Ed.). (2012). *Multiple sclerosis: A focus on rehabilitation* (5th ed.). New York, NY: National Multiple Sclerosis Society.

Kerns, R., Kassirer, M., & Otis, J. (2002). Pain in multiple sclerosis: A biopsychosocial perspective. *Journal of Rehabilitation Research and Development, 39*(2), 222–232.

Kerns, R. D., Rosenberg, R., & Otis, J. D. (2002). Self-appraised problem solving and pain-relevant social support as predictors of the experience of chronic pain. *Annals of Behavioral Medicine, 24*, 100–105. http://doi.org/10.1207/S15324796ABM2402_06

Kinsinger, S. W., Lattie, E., & Mohr, D. C. (2010). Relationship between depression, fatigue, subjective cognitive impairment, and objective neuropsychological functioning in patients with multiple sclerosis. *Neuropsychology, 24*(5), 573–580. http://doi.org/10.1037/a0019222

Koch, M., Uyttenboogaart, M., Van Harten, A., Heerings, M., & De Keyser, J. (2008). Fatigue, depression and progression in multiple sclerosis. *Multiple Sclerosis, 14*(6), 815–822. http://doi.org/10.1177/1352458508088937

Koch, M. W., Patten, S., Berzins, S., Zhornitsky, S., Greenfield, J., Wall, W., & Metz, L. M. (2014). Depression in multiple sclerosis: A long-term longitudinal study. *Multiple Sclerosis Journal, 21*(1), 78–82.

Korostil, M., & Feinstein, A. (2007). Anxiety disorders and their clinical correlates in multiple sclerosis patients. *Multiple Sclerosis, 13*(1), 67–72. http://doi.org/10.1177/1352458506071161

Kratz, A., Hirsch, A., Ehde, D., & Jensen, M. (2013). Acceptance of pain in neurological disorders: Associations with functioning and psychosocial well-being. *Rehabilitation Psychology, 55*(1), 1–9. http://doi.org/10.1037/a0031727

Kroenke, C. H., Rosner, B., Chen, W. Y., Kawachi, I., Colditz, G. A., & Holmes, M. D. (2004). Functional impact of breast cancer by age at diagnosis. *Journal of Clinical Oncology, 22*(10), 1849–1856. http://doi.org/10.1200/JCO.2004.04.173

Krupp, L. B., Christodoulou, C., Melville, P., Scherl, W. F., MacAllister, W. S., & Elkins, L. E. (2004). Donepezil improved memory in multiple sclerosis in a randomized clinical trial. *Neurology, 63*(9), 1579–1585. http://doi.org/10.1212/01.WNL.0000142989.09633.5A

Lazarus, R., & Folkman, S. (1984). *Stress, appraisal and coping*. New York, NY: Springer.

Leary, S. M. (2007). Primary-progressive multiple sclerosis. *The Lancet Neurology, 6*(10), 903–912. http://doi.org/10.1016/S1474-4422(07)70243-0

Lewinsohn, P. M. (1974). A behavioral approach to depression. In R. J. Friedman & M. M. Katz (Eds.), *The psychology of depression: Contemporary theory and research* (pp. 157–178). Oxford, UK: John Wiley & Sons.

Livneh, H., & Martz, E. (2012). Adjustment to chronic illness and disabilities: Theoretical perspectives, empirical findings, and unresolved issues. In P. Kennedy (Ed.), *The Oxford handbook of rehabilitation psychology* (pp. 47–87). New York, NY: Oxford Press.

Loring, D.W. (1999). *INS dictionary of neuropsychology*. New York, NY: Oxford University Press.

Lublin, F. D., & Reingold, S. C. (1996). Defining the clinical course of multiple sclerosis results of an international survey. *Neurology, 46*(4), 907–911. http://doi.org/10.1212/WNL.46.4.907

Lublin, F. D., Baier, M., & Cutter, G. (2003). Effect of relapses on development of residual deficit in multiple sclerosis. *Neurology, 61*(11), 1528–1532. http://doi.org/10.1212/01.WNL.0000096175.39831.21

Lublin, F. D., Reingold, S. C., Cohen, J. A. (2014). Defining the clinical course of multiple sclerosis. *Neurology, 83*(3), 278–286.

Maguire, B. L. (1996). The effects of imagery on attitudes and moods in multiple sclerosis patients. *Alternative Therapies in Health and Medicine, 2*(5), 75–79.

Maloni, H. (2003). *Multiple sclerosis and pain*. Retrieved from http://www.va.gov/MS/articles/Multiple_Sclerosis_Pain.asp

Marrie, R. A., Cohen, J., Stuve, O., Trojano, M., Sørensen, P. S., Reingold, S., & Reider, N. (2015). A systematic review of the incidence and prevalence of comorbidity in multiple sclerosis: Overview. *Multiple Sclerosis, 21*(3), 263–281. http://doi.org/10.1177/1352458514564487

McDaniel, S., Hepworth, J., & Doherty, W. J. (1992). *Medical family therapy: A biopsychosocial approach*. New York, NY: Harper Collins.

McDonald, W. I., Compston, A., Edan, G., Goodkin, D., Hartung, H. P., Lublin, F. D., & Wolinsky, J. S. (2001). Recommended diagnostic criteria for multiple sclerosis: Guidelines from the International Panel on the Diagnosis of Multiple Sclerosis. *Annals of Neurology, 50*(1), 121–127. http://doi.org/10.1002/ana.1032

McGuiness, S. (1996). Learned helplessness in the multiple sclerosis population. *Journal of Neuroscience Nursing, 28*(3), 163–170. http://doi.org/10.1097/01376517-199606000-00004

Meade, M., & Cronin, L. (2012). The expert patient and the self-management of chronic conditions and disabilities. In P. Kennedy (Ed.), *The Oxford handbook of rehabilitation psychology* (pp. 492–510). New York, NY: Oxford Press.

Melzack, R., (1975). The McGill pain questionnaire: major properties and scoring methods. *Pain, 1*(3), 227–299.

Meyer, I. H. (1995). Minority stress and mental health in gay men. *Journal of Health and Social Behavior, 36*(1), 38–56. http://doi.org/10.2307/2137286

Miller, S. (1991). Monitoring and blunting in the face of threat: Implications for adaptation and health. In L. Montada, S. Filipp, & M. Lerner (Eds.), *Life crises and experiences of loss in adulthood* (pp. 255–273). Englewood Cliffs, NJ: Erlbaum.

Miller, D. H., & Leary, S. M. (2007). Primary-progressive multiple sclerosis. *Lancet Neurology, 6,* 903–912.

Milo, R., & Miller, A. (2014). Revised diagnostic criteria of multiple sclerosis. *Autoimmunity Reviews, 13*(4), 518–524. http://doi.org/10.1016/j.autrev.2014.01.012

Minden, S. L., Feinstein, A., Kalb, R.C., Miller, D., Mohr, D.C., Patten, S. B., & Narayanaswami, P. (2014). Evidence-based guideline: Assessment and management of psychiatric disorders in individuals with MS: Report of the Guideline Development Subcommittee of the American Academy of Neurology. *Neurology, 18*(2), 174–181. http://doi.org/10.1212/WNL.0000000000000013

Minden, S. L., & Schiffer, R. B. (1990). Affective disorders in multiple sclerosis review and recommendations for clinical research. *Archives of Neurology, 47*(1), 98–104. http://doi.org/10.1001/archneur.1990.00530010124031

Mohr, D. (2007). Stress and multiple sclerosis. *Journal of Neurology, 254*(2), 1165–1168. http://doi.org/10.1007/s00415-007-2015-4

Mohr, D., Lovera, J., Brown T., Cohen, B., Neylan, T., Henry, R., Siddique, J., … Pelletier, D. (2012). A randomized trial of stress management for the prevention of new brain lesions in MS. *Neurology, 79*(5), 412–419. http://doi.org/10.1212/WNL.0b013e3182616ff9

Mohr, D. C., Boudewyn, A. C., Goodkin, D. E., Bostrom, A., & Epstein, L. (2001). Comparative outcomes for individual cognitive-behavioral therapy, supportive-expressive group therapy, and sertraline in the treatment for depression in multiple sclerosis. *Journal of Consulting and Clinical Psychology, 69*(6), 942–949. http://doi.org/10.1037/0022-006X.69.6.942

Mohr, D. C., & Cox, D. (2001). Multiple sclerosis: Empirical literature for the clinical health psychologist. *Journal of Clinical Psychology, 57*(4), 479–499. http://doi.org/10.1002/jclp.1042

Mohr, D. C., Cox, D., Epstein, L., & Boudewyn, A. (2002). Teaching patients to self-inject: Pilot study of a treatment for injection anxiety and phobia in multiple sclerosis patients prescribed injectable medications. *Journal of Behavior Therapy and Experimental Psychiatry, 33*(1), 39–47. http://doi.org/10.1016/S0005-7916(02)00011-3

Mohr, D. C., Dick, L. P., Russo, D., Pinn, J., Boudewyn, A. C., Likosky, W., & Goodkin, D. E. (1999). The psychosocial impact of multiple sclerosis: Exploring the patient's perspective. *Health Psychology, 18*(4), 376–382. http://doi.org/10.1037/0278-6133.18.4.376

Mohr, D. C., Epstein, L., Luks, T. L., Goodkin, D., Cox, D., Goldberg, A., & Nelson, S. (2003). Brain lesion volume and neuropsychological function predict efficacy of treatment for depression in multiple sclerosis. *Journal of Consulting and Clinical Psychology, 71*(6), 1017–1024. http://doi.org/10.1037/0022-006X.71.6.1017

Mohr, D. C., Goodkin, D. E., Likosky, W., Beutler, L., Gatto, N., & Langan, M. K. (1997). Identification of Beck Depression Inventory items related to multiple sclerosis. *Journal of Behavioral Medicine, 20*(4), 407–414. http://doi.org/10.1023/A:1025573315492

Mohr, D. C., Hart, S., Julian, L., Cox, D., & Pelletier, D. (2004) Association between stressful life events and exacerbation in multiple sclerosis: a meta-analysis. *British Medical Journal, 328*(7442), 731–733. http://doi.org/10.1136/bmj.38041.724421.55

Mohr, D. C., Hart, S. L., Julian, L., & Tasch, E. S. (2007). Screening for depression among patients with multiple sclerosis: Two questions may be enough. *Multiple Sclerosis, 13*(2), 215–219. http://doi.org/10.1177/1352458506070926

Mohr, D. C., Likosky, W., Bergtagnolli, A., Goodkin, D. E., Van Der Wender, J., Dwyer, P., & Dick, L. P. (2000). Telephone-administered cognitive-behavioral therapy for the treatment of depressive symptoms in multiple sclerosis. *Journal of Counseling and Clinical Psychology, 68*(2), 356–361. http://doi.org/10.1037/0022-006X.68.2.356

MS Society of Canada. (2008). *Pain and MS.* Retrieved from http://mssociety.ca/en/pdf/managing-ms-pain.pdf

National Center for Complementary and Integrative Health (NCCIH). (n.d.). *Complementary, alternative, or integrative health: What's in a name?* Retrieved from https://nccih.nih.gov/health/integrative-health

National Multiple Sclerosis Society. (2012). *Multiple Scleroris: A focus on rehabilitation* (5th ed.). New York, NY: Professional Resource Center NMSS.

Nordin, L., & Rorsman, I. (2012). Cognitive behavioural therapy in multiple sclerosis: A randomized controlled pilot study of acceptance and commitment therapy. *Journal of Rehabilitation Medicine, 44*, 87–90. http://doi.org/10.2340/16501977-0898

Noy, S., Achiron, A., Gabbay, U., Barak, Y., Rotstein, Z., Laor, N., & Sarova-Pinhas, I. (1995). A new approach to affective symptoms in relapsing-remitting multiple sclerosis. *Comprehensive Psychiatry, 36*(5), 390–395. http://doi.org/10.1016/S0010-440X(95)90121-3

Nyenhuis, D. L., Rao, S. M., Zajecka, J. M., Luchetta, T., Bernardin, L., & Garron, D. C. (1995). Mood disturbance versus other symptoms of depression in multiple sclerosis. *Journal of the International Neuropsychological Society, 1*(03), 291–296. http://doi.org/10.1017/S135561770000028X

Oken, B. S., Kishiyama, S., Zajdel, D., Bourdette, D., Carlsen, J., Haas, M., … & Mass, M. (2004) Randomized controlled trial of yoga and exercise in multiple sclerosis. *Neurology, 62*(11), 2058–2064.

Olkin, R. (1999). *What psychotherapists should know about disability.* New York, NY: The Guilford Press.

Olkin, R. (2009). Disability-affirmative therapy. In I. Marini & M. Stebnicki (Eds.), *The professional counselor's desk reference* (pp. 355–369). New York, NY: Springer.

Olsen, S. A. (2009). A review of complementary and alternative medicine (CAM) by people with multiple sclerosis. *Occupational Therapy International, 16*(1), 57–70. http://doi.org/10.1002/oti.266

Ontaneda, D., & Rae-Grant, A. D. (2009). Management of acute exacerbations in multiple sclerosis. *Annals of Indian Academy of Neurology, 12*(4), 264. http://doi.org/10.4103/0972-2327.58283

Pakenham, K. (2012). Multiple sclerosis. In P. Kennedy (Ed.), *Oxford handbook of rehabilitation psychology* (pp. 211–244). New York, NY: Oxford Press.

Pakenham, K., & Cox, S. (2009). The dimensional structure of benefit finding in multiple sclerosis and relations with positive and negative adjustment: A longitudinal study. *Psychology and Health, 24*(4), 373–393. http://doi.org/10.1080/08870440701832592

Panitch, H., Goodin, D. S., Francis, G. F., Chang, P., Coyle, P. K., O'Connor, P., & Weinshenker, B. (2002). Randomized, comparative study of interferon β-1a treatment regimens in MS: The Evidence Trial. *Neurology, 59*(10), 1496–1506. http://doi.org/10.1212/01.WNL.0000034080.43681.DA

Paparrigopoulos, T., Ferentinos, P., Kouzoupis, A., Koutsis, G., & Papadimitriou, G. N. (2010). The neuropsychiatry of multiple sclerosis: Focus on disorders of mood, affect and behaviour. *International Review of Psychiatry, 22*(1), 14–21. http://doi.org/10.3109/09540261003589323

Pargament, K. I. (1997). *The psychology of religion and coping.* New York, NY: Guilford.

Pargament, K. I., Smith, B. W., Koenig, H. G., & Perez, L. (1998). Patterns of positive and negative religious coping with major life stressors. *Journal for the Scientific Study of Religion, 37,* 710–724. http://doi.org/10.2307/1388152

Patti, F. (2010). Optimizing the benefit of multiple sclerosis therapy: The importance of treatment adherence. *Patient Preference and Adherence, 4,* 1–9. http://doi.org/10.2147/PPA.S8230

Pepping, M., & Ehde, D. M. (2005). Neuropsychological evaluation and treatment of multiple sclerosis: The importance of a neuro-rehabilitation focus. *Physical Medicine and Rehabilitation Clinics of North America, 16*(2), 411–436. http://doi.org/10.1016/j.pmr.2005.01.009

Persons, J. B., & Davidson, J. (2010). Cognitive-behavioral case formulation. In K. Dobson (Ed.), *Handbook of cognitive-behavioral therapies* (3rd ed., pp. 172–196). New York, NY: Guilford.

Peterson, C., & Seligman, M. E. P. (1987). Explanatory style and illness. *Journal of Personality, 55,* 237–265. doi: 10.1111/j.1467-6494.1987.tb00436.x

Phillips, M. (2007). *Reversing chronic pain.* Berkeley, CA: North Atlantic Books.

Phillips, M., & Frederick, C. (1995). *Healing the divided self: Clinical and Ericksonian hypnotherapy for post-traumatic and dissociative conditions.* New York, NY: Norton.

Phillips, M., & Levine, P. (2012). *Freedom from pain: Discover your body's power to overcome physical pain.* Boulder, CO: Sounds True.

Porcel, J., Río, J., Sánchez-Betancourt, A., Arévalo, M. J., Tintoré, M., Téllez, N., Borràs, C. ... Montalbán, X. (2006). Long-term emotional state of multiple sclerosis patients treated with interferon beta. *Multiple Sclerosis, 12*(6), 802–807. http://doi.org/10.1177/1352458506070748

Porges, S. W. (2001) The polyvagal theory: Phylogenetic substrates of a social nervous system. *International Journal of Psychophysiology, 42*(2), 123–146. Retrieved from http://wisebrain.org/PolyvagalTheory.pdf

Rao, S. M., Leo, G. J., Bernardin, L., & Unverzagt, F. (1991). Cognitive dysfunction in multiple sclerosis. I. Frequency, patterns, and prediction. *Neurology, 41*(5), 685–691. http://doi.org/10.1212/WNL.41.5.685

Reitman, N., & Kalb, R. (2012). *Multiple sclerosis: A model of psychosocial support* (5th ed.). New York, NY: Professional Resource Center, National MS Society.

Renoux, C., Vukusic, S., Mikaeloff, Y., Edan, G., Clanet, M., Dubois, B., & Confavreux, C. (2007). Natural history of multiple sclerosis with childhood onset. *New England Journal of Medicine, 356*(25), 2603–2613. http://doi.org/10.1056/NEJMoa067597

Rocky Mountain MS Center. (n.d.). *Alternative medicine, wellness, and diet.* Retrieved from http://www.mscenter.org/resources/publications

Rutter, M. (1985). Resilience is the face of adversity. Protective factors and resistance to psychiatric disorder. *British Journal of Psychiatry, 147,* 598–561. http://doi.org/10.1192/bjp.147.6.598

Sá, M. J. (2008). Psychological aspects of multiple sclerosis. *Clinical Neurology and Neurosurgery, 110*(9), 868–877. http://doi.org/10.1016/j.clineuro.2007.10.001

Schiffer, R. B., Wineman, N. M., & Weitkamp, L. R. (1986). Association between bipolar affective disorder and multiple sclerosis. *American Journal of Psychiatry, 143,* 94–95. http://doi.org/10.1176/ajp.143.1.94

Schiffer, R. B., & Wineman, N. M. (1990). Antidepressant pharmacotherapy of depression. *American Journal of Psychiatry, 147*(1), 1493–1497. http://doi.org/10.1176/ajp.147.11.1493

Schwartz, C. E., Coulthart-Morris, L., & Zeng, Q. (1996). Psychosocial correlates of fatigue in multiple sclerosis. *Archives Physical Medicine Rehabilitation, 77*(2), 165–170. http://doi.org/10.1016/S0003-9993(96)90162-8

Schwartz, C. E., & Rogers, M. (1994). Designing a psychosocial intervention to teach coping flexibility. *Rehabilitation Psychology, 39*(1), 57–72. http://doi.org/10.1037/h0080312

Schwarzer, R., Dunkel-Schetter, C., & Kemeny, M. (1994). The multidimensional nature of received social support in gay men at risk of HIV infection and AIDS. *American Journal of Community Psychology, 22*(3), 319–339. http://doi.org/10.1007/BF02506869

Schwarzer, R., Knoll, N., & Reickmann, N. (2003). Social support. In A. Kaptein & J. Weinman (Eds.), *Introduction to health psychology* (pp. 158–181). Oxford, UK: Blackwell.

Seligman, M. E. P., & Czikszentmihalyi, M. (2000). Positive psychology. *American Psychologist, 55*(1), 5–14. http://doi.org/10.1037/0003-066X.55.1.5

Senders, A., Wahbeh, H., Spain, R., & Shinto, L. (2012). Mind-body medicine for multiple sclerosis: A systematic review (abstract). *Autoimmune Disorders*, 2012, Article ID 567324, 12 pp. http://doi.org/10.1155/2012/567324

Serafini, B., Rosicarelli, B., Franciotta, D., Magliozzi, R., Reynolds, R., Cinque, P., & Aloisi, F. (2007). Dysregulated Epstein-Barr virus infection in the multiple sclerosis brain. *The Journal of Experimental Medicine, 204*(12), 2899–2912. http://doi.org/10.1084/jem.20071030

Sheppard, S. C., Forsyth, J. P., Hickling, E. J., & Bianchi, J. (2010). A novel application of acceptance and commitment therapy for psychosocial problems associated with multiple sclerosis: Results from a half-day workshop intervention. *International Journal of MS Care, 12*(4), 200–206. http://doi.org/10.7224/1537-2073-12.4.200

Sidhom, Y., Ben Djebara, M., Hizem, Y., Abdelkefi, I., Kacem, I., Gargouri, A., & Gouider, R. (2014). Bipolar disorder and multiple sclerosis: A case series. *Behavioural Neurology, 2014*, 1–4. http://doi.org/10.1155/2014/536503

Simpson, S., Blizzard, L., Otahal, P., Van der Mei, I., & Taylor, B. (2011). Latitude is significantly associated with the prevalence of multiple sclerosis: A meta-analysis. *Journal of Neurology, Neurosurgery & Psychiatry, 82*(10), 1132–1141. http://doi.org/10.1136/jnnp.2011.240432

Simpson, R., Booth, J. Lawrence, M., Byrne, S., Mair, F., & Mercer, S. (2014). Mindfulness based interventions in multiple sclerosis: A systematic review. *BMC Neurology, 14*(15). http://doi.org/10.1186/1471-2377-14-15

Smedema, S., Bakken-Gillen, S., & Dalton, J. (2009) Psychosocial adaptation to chronic illness and disability: Models and measurement. In F. Chan, E. Cardosa, & J. Chronister (Eds.), *Understanding psychosocial adjustment to chronic illness and disability* (pp. 51–71). New York, NY: Springer.

Stone, J., Reuber, M., & Carson, A. (2013). Functional symptoms in neurology: Mimics and chameleons. *Practical Neurology, 13*(2), 104–113. http://doi.org/10.1136/practneurol-2012-000422

Strober, L. B., & Arnett, P. A. (2010). Assessment of depression in multiple sclerosis: Development of a "trunk and branch" model. *The Clinical Neuropsychologist, 24*(7), 1146–1166. http://doi.org/10.1080/13854046.2010.514863

Sue, D. (2010). *Microaggressions in everyday life: Race, gender and sexual orientation.* Hoboken, NJ: Wiley.

Suls, J., & Fletcher, B. (1985). The relative efficacy of avoidant and nonavoidant coping strategies: A meta-analysis. *Health Psychology, 4*(3), 249–288. http://doi.org/10.1037/0278-6133.4.3.249

Taber, K. H., Hurley, R. A., & Yudofsky, S. C. (2010). Diagnosis and treatment of neuropsychiatric disorders. *Annual Review of Medicine, 61*, 121–133. http://doi.org/10.1146/annurev.med.051408.105018

Thomas, P. W., Thomas, S., Hillier, C., Galvin, K., & Baker, R. (2006). Psychological interventions for multiple sclerosis. In P. W. Thomas (Ed.), *Cochrane Database of Systematic Reviews* (1), CD004431. http://doi.org/10.1002/14651858.CD004431.pub2

Tintoré, M., Rovira, A., Rio, J., Nos, C., Grive, E., Tellez, N., & Montalban, X. (2006). Baseline MRI predicts future attacks and disability in clinically isolated syndromes. *Neurology, 67*(6), 968–972. http://doi.org/10.1212/01.wnl.0000237354.10144.ec

Wahbeh, H., Elsas, S.-M., & Oken, B. (2008). Mind–body interventions: Applications in neurology. *Neurology, 70*(24), 2321–2328. http://doi.org/10.1212/01.wnl.0000314667.16386.5e

Wainapel, S., & Fast, A. (2003). *Alternative medicine and rehabilitation – a guide for practitioners.* New York, NY: Demos Medical Publishing.

Weisbrot, D., Charvet, L., Serafin, D., Milazzo, M., Preston, T., Cleary, R., & Krupp, L. (2014). Psychiatric diagnoses and cognitive impairment in pediatric multiple sclerosis. *Multiple Sclerosis, 20*(5), 588–593. http://doi.org/10.1177/1352458513504249

Wilken, J. A., & Sullivan, C. (2007). Recognizing and treating common psychiatric disorders in multiple sclerosis. *The Neurologist, 13*(6), 343–354. http://doi.org/10.1097/NRL.0b013e31806dc2e8

Williams-Piehota, P., Pizarro, J., Schneider, T. R., Mowad, L., & Salovey, P. (2005). Matching health messages to monitor-blunter coping styles to motivate screening mammography. *Health Psychology, 24*(1), 58–67. http://doi.org/10.1037/0278-6133.24.1.58

Wingerchuk, D. M., & Carter, J. L. (2014). Multiple sclerosis: current and emerging disease-modifying therapies and treatment strategies. *Mayo Clinic Proceedings, 89*(2), 225–240. http://doi.org/10.1016/j.mayocp.2013.11.002

World Health Organization. (2001). *The international classification of functioning, disability and health (ICF)*. Geneva, Switzerland: Author. Retrieved from http://www.who.int/classifications/icf/en/

Wortman, C. B., & Brehm, J. W. (1975). Responses to uncontrollable outcomes: An integration of reactance theory and the learned helplessness model. In L. Berkowitz (Ed.), *Advances in experimental social psychology* (Vol. 8, pp. 277–336). New York, NY: Academic Press. http://dx.doi.org/10.1016/s0065-2601(08)60253-1

Yeh, E. A., & Weinstock-Guttman, B. (2012). The management of pediatric multiple sclerosis. *Journal of Child Neurology, 27*(11), 1384–1393. http://doi.org/10.1177/0883073812452785

Zankowski, S. G., Hall, M. H., Klein, L. C., & Baum, A. (2001). Appraised control, coping, and stress in a community sample: A test of the goodness-of-fit hypothesis. *Annals of Behavioral Medicine, 23*(3), 158–165. http://doi.org/10.1207/S15324796ABM2303_3

8

Appendix: Tools and Resources

Clinical Interview – Focus on MS

Key considerations in working with individuals with MS:

Accessibility: Assess alternative transportation, access to office stairs, ramp, disability restrooms, and parking, contractual arrangements regarding psychotherapy practice (e.g., considering not implementing typical fee if missed appointment without client providing prior notice); assess comfort of office (e.g., temperature, seating).

Neurologic and Treatment History: Relationship with neurologist and primary care doctor; MS symptoms; onset, course, when diagnosed with MS; experience of being diagnosed/prior to diagnosis; abilities and disabilities; past and present treatment successes and failures; their understanding of their diagnosis; treatment engagement issues.

Physical Symptom Current Impact, Onset, Treatment, Outcomes: Physical symptoms (such as fatigue, pain, spasticity, reduced mobility, bowel/bladder dysfunction, sexual health) and their impact on day-to-day life, relationships, psychological well-being.

Consult: Consider consultation with neurologist and other medical providers to verify diagnostic information and medical history.

Impact on Adaptive Functioning: Self-care: eating, sleeping, exercise, work habits, ability to manage daily living skills (basic, such as dressing, bathing and more advanced, such as finances and healthcare management).

Work-Related Issues: Current occupational functioning and job security, need for accommodation and desire or need to exit or re-enter work world.

Interpersonal Functioning: Relationships with family, friends, significant others; perceptions of others, such as misattributing attention problems for disinterest, or invalidating the impact of "invisible" symptoms (e.g., fatigue, pain, mood disturbance, cognitive dysfunction).

Illness Perceptions: How client (and those who raised him or her) dealt with common childhood illness and accidents. This may be reflected in how a client responds to his or her MS symptoms.

Substance Use: Drug, alcohol, food, and other substance abuse. This includes a full assessment of how a client is using prescribed medication and avoidance style coping.

Coping Skills: Past successes, challenges, and coping tools,

Resources: Current and past connections to MS community resources, such as support groups, MS-related organization, and/or disability rights organizations.

Rehabilitation: Perception, opinion, and knowledge of rehabilitation options: neuropsychological evaluation, cognitive rehabilitation, physical therapy, occupational therapy, speech therapy, use of assistive technology, use of aids to mobility and physical functioning, use of resources to enhance independent living.

Spiritual Coping: Religious background and current spiritual belief and community.

Culture: Relationship with dominant culture – Assessment of diversity issues that may impact therapy and access to healthcare; language barriers impacting communication with healthcare professionals.

Phases of Wellness – Building a Wellness Plan

(Although this is in a linear format, it is not necessarily a linear process, with the last phase being the goal. Phases will occur out of order and need to be repeated when there is new information or changes.)

Gathering Information

A. MS and you
1. Getting a diagnosis and ongoing evaluation
2. Getting educated about your diagnosis and treatment options
3. Resources
   a. Personal
      1. Financial
      2. Time
      3. Expertise and knowledge
      4. Family and friends
         i. Who is willing and able to offer support?
         ii. Whose support is helpful to you?
         iii. Who is fun to be with?
         iv. Who causes you stress?
   b. External
      1. Societies and organizations
      2. Hospitals with special centers
      3. Expertise in your community
4. Yourself
   a. What internal resources do you have?
   b. What are your strengths?
   c. What do you enjoy doing?
   d. What makes you happy?
   e. What causes you stress?
   f. What are you willing to change for better self-care?
5. Your body (fatigue management)
   a. How much sleep do you need?
   b. When do you feel better? Worse?
   c. What times of day are best for you?
   d. What are your symptoms and abilities?
   e. How much exercise revives/exhausts you?
   f. What types of food or eating habits are best for you?
6. Work habits (paid, volunteer, or household)
   a. How many hours a week are you able to work?
   b. How many hours a day are you able to work?
   c. How often do you need breaks?
   d. What type of work is best suited to you?
   e. What type of work causes you too much stress?

B. Your care
1. Self-care
   a. Nutrition
   b. Exercise

From: P. B. Werfel, R. E. Franco Durán, and L. J. Trettin: *Multiple Sclerosis*

© 2016 Hogrefe Publishing

    c. Rest and relaxation

    d. Balance and pacing

2. Professional healthcare – building a comprehensive treatment team

    a. What treatments are available?

    b. How effective are they?

    c. What are the side effects?

    d. How much does it cost?

    e. Where do I get referrals?

    f. How much experience does the professional have with MS?

    g. Do your healthcare providers listen to you and take your concerns seriously?

3. Western medicine

    a. Medication

    b. Physical therapy

    c. Occupational therapy

    d. Cognitive therapy

    e. Rehabilitation therapy

4. Complementary and alternative medicine

    a. Resources

        1. Rocky Mountain MS Center (http://livingwell.mscenter.org)

        2. http://www.neurologycare.net/cam

5. Mind–body interventions

    a. Imagery/hypnosis

    b. Mindfulness/meditation

    c. Breathing and relaxation techniques

    d. Biofeedback

5. Other healing avenues

    a. Psychotherapy

    b. Yoga, tai chi, qi gong, other movements

    c. Support groups

Realization and Acceptance

    A. No shame, no blame. You didn't cause MS.

    B. How can you make living with MS easier for you?

    C. You are still you. Focus on what is meaningful in your life.

    D. Discover ways to adjust and adapt

    E. Focus on what you CAN do.

Honoring Feelings

    A. You will experience a range of emotions.

    B. Allow yourself some time to explore them.

    C. Grief, anger, sadness, and frustration are expectable but seek help for depression and anxiety.

    D. Share your feelings with safe and compassionate others.

    E. Be willing to seek help from a professional

Connection–Community

    A. Connection with people: Talk with people who have the same or similar diagnoses. Talk with friends and family. Participate in social activities.

From: P. B. Werfel, R. E. Franco Durán, and L. J. Trettin: *Multiple Sclerosis*

© 2016 Hogrefe Publishing

B. Connection with spirit: If religion or spirituality is part of your life, seek support and strength there. Prayer can help with stress reduction.

C. Connection with community: You are part of a larger community and you have something to offer. Get involved to any extent that you can and stay involved.

Initial Adjustment

A. Based on the information you have gathered and your support network, you will be able to develop and implement an initial wellness plan.

B. This plan is unique to you and will need to be amended as your needs or circumstances change.

Anticipated Sabotage

A. Expect that there will be times when you don't want to think about health, MS, self-care, or wellness.

B. When things are going well you may want to forget that you have MS and stop helpful activities or treatments.

C. If symptoms increase, you may become disillusioned and feel like nothing will help.

D. This is not the time to stop helping yourself. This is time to reassess.

Reassessment

A. Amend your wellness plan to more closely align with your needs and lifestyle.

B. If you have taken on more than is realistic, determine what treatments and self-care activities are the most useful and discuss a modification with your healthcare providers.

C. If your symptoms have changed, you may need to explore different therapies that may increase your health and wellness.

Living and Thriving

A. You take actions that will enable you to live better with MS.

B. You have a wellness plan that you feel confident in.

C. You have a team of healthcare providers that you trust.

D. You are willing to make changes that will maximize your abilities.

E. You have become more realistic and compassionate with yourself.

F. You have the supportive relationships

From: P. B. Werfel, R. E. Franco Durán, and L. J. Trettin: *Multiple Sclerosis*   © 2016 Hogrefe Publishing

Helping Clients to Evaluate Coping Strategies

Strategy	Elements	Benefits	Difficulties
Avoidant	Distraction	Decreases stress in the short-term, helpful with acute symptoms	Prevents problem solving, does not address situation or increase wellness
Psychological	Exploring feelings and emotions	Can allow for reframing, acceptance, and psychological adjustment	Can increase distress, lead to helplessness, and deter problem solving
Instrumental/problem-focused	Problem solving, taking action, doing it differently	Address the issue, increase self-mastery and management	May increase distress if utilized to avoid rather than address emotional distress; May result in pressure to "do something"
Meaning-focused	Finding life's lessons, making lemonade out of lemons	Strengthening relationships, personal and spiritual growth	Can prevent helpful action
Benefit finding	Positive reframing, prayer, reorganizing priorities	Increases acceptance and decreases distress	Can prevent helpful action and produce pressure to always "look on the bright side"

From: P. B. Werfel, R. E. Franco Durán, and L. J. Trettin: *Multiple Sclerosis*   © 2016 Hogrefe Publishing

Pain History

Briefly describe pain history (significant events, the approximate dates of those events, and physicians and hospitals):

_____

_____

_____

_____

_____

_____

_____

_____

Treatment History:

Surgery
Dates	Surgeon	Was it helpful?
_____	_____	Yes _____ No _____
_____	_____	Yes _____ No _____

Nerve Blocks
Dates	Physician	Was it helpful?
_____	_____	Yes _____ No _____

Steroid injection
Dates	Physician	Was it helpful?
_____	_____	Yes _____ No _____
_____	_____	Yes _____ No _____

Physical Therapy
Dates	Where	Was it helpful?
_____	_____	Yes _____ No _____
_____	_____	Yes _____ No _____

TNS Unit
Dates	Where	Was it helpful?
_____	_____	Yes _____ No _____

Psychological (relaxation, biofeedback, multidisciplinary)
Dates	Therapist	Was it helpful?
_____	_____	Yes _____ No _____

Chiropractic
Dates	Where	Was it helpful?
_____	_____	Yes _____ No _____

From: P. B. Werfel, R. E. Franco, and L. J. Trettin: *Multiple Sclerosis*   © 2016 Hogrefe Publishing

Pain medications past and current:

Medication	Dates	Dosage	Helpful?
_____	_____	_____	Yes _____ No _____
_____	_____	_____	Yes _____ No _____
_____	_____	_____	Yes _____ No _____
_____	_____	_____	Yes _____ No _____
_____	_____	_____	Yes _____ No _____
_____	_____	_____	Yes _____ No _____
_____	_____	_____	Yes _____ No _____
_____	_____	_____	Yes _____ No _____

What makes your pain better? worse? no effect?

	Better	Worse	No effect
Heat	_____	_____	_____
Cold	_____	_____	_____
Bath/shower	_____	_____	_____
Walking	_____	_____	_____
Sitting	_____	_____	_____
Lying down/sleeping	_____	_____	_____
Stress/worry	_____	_____	_____
Exercise/activity	_____	_____	_____
Sexual activity	_____	_____	_____
Reading/television	_____	_____	_____

Pain Pattern:

_____ continuous   _____ comes and goes   _____ brief/momentary

WORSE during a certain time of the day?
        If yes, when? _____

BETTER during a certain time of the day?
        If yes, when? _____

Pain intensity:
Circle the appropriate number: 0 = *no pain*, and 10 = *worst pain imaginable*

AVERAGE pain: 0 1 2 3 4 5 6 7 8 9 10

MINIMUM pain: 0 1 2 3 4 5 6 7 8 9 10

MAXIMUM pain: 0 1 2 3 4 5 6 7 8 9 10

Description of Current Pain:

Symbols:

- - - -	o o o o	x x x x	/ / / /	+ + + +
numbness	pins/needles	burning	stabbing	aching

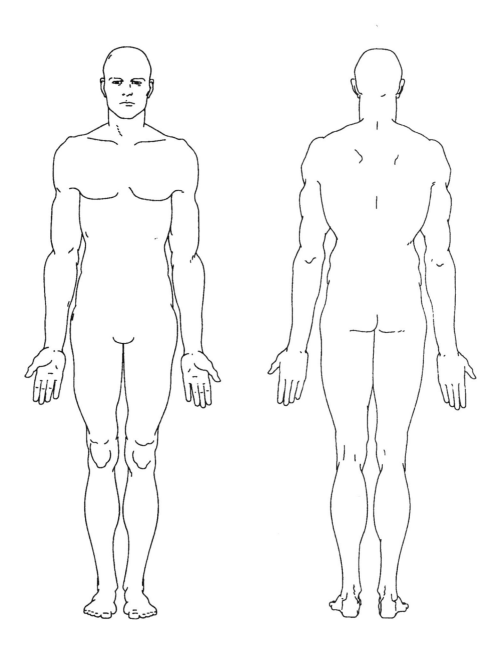

From: P. B. Werfel, R. E. Franco, and L. J. Trettin: *Multiple Sclerosis*   © 2016 Hogrefe Publishing

Some Questions to Ask to Evaluate the Use of Pain Medication

- Is more than one physician prescribing pain medication for you?
- How often do you speak with your physician about your discomfort and your use of medication?
- Do you sometimes take more than prescribed or in shorter intervals?
- Do you take your pain medication when you are upset about something?
- Do you combine your medication with alcohol?
- Do you take pain medications even when you are not in pain or because of fear of discomfort?
- Is your pain medication effective in decreasing your pain?
- Do you hesitate to use the medication as prescribed because of side effects?

From: P. B. Werfel, R. E. Franco Durán, and L. J. Trettin: *Multiple Sclerosis*   © 2016 Hogrefe Publishing

Peer Commentaries

Multiple sclerosis is one of the most terrifying and challenging diseases to treat. The three authors of the newly released book, Multiple Sclerosis, *manage to cover an enormous amount of material in a comprehensive and highly practical format. They begin by specifying definitions and different versions of the disease, medical and psychological symptoms, related diagnoses, and neurological difficulties. Particularly useful are the chapters on diagnostic complexity and treatment approaches, which include topics such as stress and pain management, learned helplessness, focus of psychotherapy, medical and alternative treatments, and mind-body approaches and group interventions. The volume closes with three case vignettes. This book should be on the desks of psychiatrists, psychologists, and all mental health and medical health providers. If it had been available when I was diagnosing and treating my first MS patient, I have no doubt that my efficacy and the patient's outcome would have been exponentially improved! I highly recommend this integrative work.*

Maggie Phillips, PhD, private practice, Oakland, CA; Author of *Healing the Divided Self* (with Claire Frederick, MD), *Finding the Energy to Heal*, *Reversing Chronic Pain*, and *Freedom From Pain* (with Dr. Peter Levine)

Multiple sclerosis is a lifelong disorder which commonly begins in early adult years and the effects and long-term course of which vary enormously from one individual to another. Whether its manifestations are minimal or severely disabling, MS may cause huge uncertainty about the future, especially in young adults who are just getting established in their occupations and starting their families. This uncertainty, along with the fact that very common symptoms of MS such as pathological fatigue, depression, and subtle cognitive change are invisible to others, presents very unique challenges to behavioral health providers. This book provides an excellent guided tour into the type of symptoms and long-term course of MS as well as medical background relating to diagnosis and treatment. These important tools will help any mental health professional provide better care for those with multiple sclerosis.

John Schafer, MD, FAAN, Director, Mercy MS Center, Sacramento, CA; Medical Director MS Achievement Center, Citrus Heights, CA

As a young psychologist starting to see patients with multiple sclerosis (MS) more than thirty years ago, I had the opportunity to learn about the disease from a gifted interdisciplinary team of MS experts. But I had no roadmap for addressing the complex emotional, cognitive, and psychosocial challenges faced by individuals living with MS and their families. My patients were kind enough to teach me what I needed to know, but I am sure they would have preferred for me to come prepared with the wealth of information provided by Drs. Werfel, Durán, and Trettin. These authors have used their shared wealth of experience and expertise to ground the reader in the medical, psychiatric, psychological, and social aspects of MS, while bringing the realities of this disease to life through case vignettes. The information is comprehensive yet accessible, with clinical pearls, clear definitions, and tables for quick reference. This book is an essential resource for any mental health professional involved in the care of individuals affected by MS.

Rosalind Kalb, PhD, Vice President, Healthcare Information & Resources, Advocacy, Services and Research Department, National Multiple Sclerosis Society, New York, NY; Author of *Multiple Sclerosis: The Questions you Have – The Answers you Need, Multiple Sclerosis For Dummies,* and *Multiple Sclerosis: A Focus on Rehabilitation*

This book is the one-stop shop for information about multiple sclerosis. From the lay-out of the table of contents to the helpful tables to the margin notes with key points, the book is clear, concise, and comprehensive. The explanation of MS and its symptoms will be useful for members of the treatment team, whether they are professionals (e.g., therapists) or family members. The emphasis on the idiosyncrasy of the disorder, as well as the cultural and contextual variables for the person with MS, makes it clear that treatment cannot be one-size-fits-all. The inclusion of clinical vignettes and different ways of conceptualizing a chronic illness or disability such as MS is a valuable tool for therapists to use in understanding their clients' perspectives on their MS. I particularly liked the integration of medical aspects with psychosocial variables, leading to a well-rounded discussion of the experiences of persons with MS. Although some books on MS can be overwhelming for someone who is newly diagnosed, this version is straightforward and non-threatening, as it matter-of-factly includes all possible symptoms and many variants of medical and psychosocial treatment. The appendices include a guide for clinical interviewing, steps in building a wellness plan, ways to evaluate coping strategies, and how to understand pain medication usage. This is the book for all those with MS, their families, and their treatment team members.

Rhoda Olkin, PhD, Distinguished Professor, California School of Professional Psychology at Alliant International University, San Francisco, CA; Author of *What Psychotherapists Should Know About Disability and Disability-Affirmative Therapy*

Multiple Sclerosis provides a great foundation for behavioral health professionals. It provides good educational material on multiple sclerosis and MS management, with more depth in areas that are not provided in other MS resources, mainly the cognitive and emotional challenges of people living with MS. The book is a resource for mental health and other healthcare professionals who work with people living with MS since the cognitive and emotional challenges are often a large component of adherence to a treatment regimen. It is a resource that would be great to have on the bookshelf of all healthcare professionals working with people diagnosed with MS.

Brian Hutchinson, PT, MSCS, Director, Dignity Health, MS Achievement Center, Citrus Heights, CA

Multiple sclerosis can affect patients and their loved ones in many ways that are sometimes challenging to manage, especially neuropsychological and psychiatric issues. The recognition of these symptoms frequently associated with the disease is key as it allows broadening the scope of patient care, to encompass all aspects of life that may be affected. This book is an outstanding resource for healthcare providers who care for patients with MS and their families.

Emmanuelle Waubant, MD, PhD, Professor of Neurology and Pediatrics, Multiple Sclerosis Center, University of California, San Francisco, CA